Ste

RADIATI
Treatmen

GW01246466

Step by Step®

RADIATION THERAPY
Treatment and Planning

Editor

Arun Kumar Rathi

MBBS (Gold Medalist) MD (Radiotherapy)

Professor of Radiotherapy
Maulana Azad Medical College and
Associated Lok Nayak Hospital, New Delhi, India

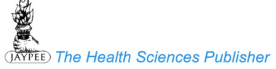

JAYPEE *The Health Sciences Publisher*

New Delhi | London | Philadelphia | Panama

Jaypee Brothers Medical Publishers (P) Ltd.

Headquarters

Jaypee Brothers Medical Publishers (P) Ltd.
4838/24, Ansari Road, Daryaganj
New Delhi 110 002, India
Phone: +91-11-43574357
Fax: +91-11-43574314
E-mail: jaypee@jaypeebrothers.com

Overseas Offices

J.P. Medical Ltd.
83, Victoria Street, London
SW1H 0HW (UK)
Phone: +44 20 3170 8910
Fax: +44 (0)20 3008 6180
E-mail: info@jpmedpub.com

Jaypee-Highlights Medical Publishers Inc.
City of Knowledge, Bld. 237, Clayton
Panama City, Panama
Phone: +1 507-301-0496
Fax: +1 507-301-0499
E-mail: cservice@jphmedical.com

Jaypee Medical Inc.
325, Chestnut Street
Suite 412, Philadelphia, PA 19106, USA
Phone: +1 267-519-9789
E-mail: jpmed.us@gmail.com

Jaypee Brothers Medical Publishers (P) Ltd.
17/1-B, Babar Road, Block-B, Shaymali
Mohammadpur, Dhaka-1207
Bangladesh
Mobile: +08801912003485
E-mail: jaypeedhaka@gmail.com

Jaypee Brothers Medical Publishers (P) Ltd.
Bhotahity, Kathmandu, Nepal
Phone: +977-9741283608
E-mail: kathmandu@jaypeebrothers.com

Website: www.jaypeebrothers.com
Website: www.jaypeedigital.com

Step by Step® Radiation Therapy: Treatment and Planning

First Edition: **2016**

ISBN: 978-93-5250-124-3

Printed at Rajkamal Electric Press, Plot No. 2, Phase-IV, Kundli, Haryana.

Contributors

Ashutosh Mukherji MD
Associate Professor
Department of Radiotherapy
Regional Cancer Center
JIPMER, Puducherry, India

Gautam Saran MD
Head and DNB Coordinator
Department of Radiation Oncology
MN Budhrani Cancer Institute
Inlaks and Budhrani Hospital
Pune, Maharashtra, India

Indu Bansal MD DHM
Senior Consultant
Department of Radiation Oncology
Max Hospital
Saket, New Delhi, India

Kanika Sharma MD
Consultant
Dharmshilla Hospital
New Delhi, India

Vikash Kumar MD
Consultant
Department of Radiation Oncology
Jaypee Hospital
Noida, Uttar Pradesh, India

Preface

This book has been written for young doctors who begin their journey in the field of Radiation Oncology. Radiation oncology is a very vast branch, and unlike other branches, students hardly get any exposure in this specialty in their MBBS curriculum. So, it is very difficult for the students to take a dip in the vast ocean and take out pearls of wisdom easily. This book is a sincere attempt to make their work easier and hence focuses on basic principles of radiation therapy planning, verification and delivery of treatment in a step-by-step manner.

When I was approached to write a book on radiotherapy planning, the first thought that came to my mind was the young learners. I immediately called five of my students, enquired about their needs and the foundation for the book was laid there and then. This book has been planned with a lot of inputs from all of them. In fact, many chapters of the book are contributed by them. I am thankful to each and every one of them. For this reason, I call this book *Step by Step Radiation Therapy: Treatment and Planning* by the residents for the residents.

I know that in spite of all the best efforts, there could still be many shortcomings in this book. I would really appreciate all your suggestions and criticism in a positive manner, and assure you of improving it further in all the future editions.

Arun Kumar Rathi

Contents

Introduction

Nearly all cancer patients receive radiation therapy as definitive therapy, for palliation or as adjunct to surgery or chemotherapy.

The aim of radiation therapy is to deliver a precisely measured dose of radiation to a defined tumor volume with minimal damage to surrounding healthy tissues.

Resulting in

- Eradication of tumor
- A high and improved quality of life
- Prolongation of survival
- Effective palliation of symptoms of cancer
- With minimal morbidity.

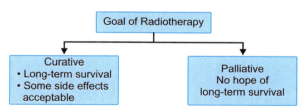

Simpler treatment techniques that yield an acceptable dose distribution are to be preferred over costly and complex ones, which have a greater margin of error in day-to-day treatment.

IMPORTANT POINTS OF ANATOMY FOR RADIATION ONCOLOGISTS

Surface anatomy is the study of deeper parts in relation to the skin surface. A mental picture of surface anatomy is needed by every doctor during the physical examination of a case and radiotherapy planning. Radiological anatomy is the study of deeper organs by plain or contrast radiography.

Breast

- Breasts vary in size.
- Normally between ribs 2 and 6, overlie the pectoralis major muscle.
- Axillary tail—superolaterally around the lower margin of pectoralis major muscle.

Thoracic Level 4/5

- Costal cartilage of rib 2 articulate with the sternum.
- Superior mediastinum separated from inferior mediastinum.
- Ascending aorta ends and arch of aorta begins.
- The trachea bifurcates.

Spinal Cord and Subarachnoid Space

Normally in adults, spinal cord terminates at the level of disc between L1 and L2. Subarachnoid space ends at approximately S2 (sacral dimples).

Vertebral Spinous Processes

C2: Most superior bony protuberance in the midline inferior to the skull.

C3-4: Upper margin of thyroid cartilage
Bifurcation of common carotid artery into internal and external carotid arteries.

C6: Transition from pharynx to esophagus
Larynx to trachea
Inferior margin of cricoid cartilage

C7: Prominent eminence in the midline at the base of the neck.

T1: Inferior to C7, visible as midline protuberance, often more prominent than the spinous process of C7.

T3: Root of the spine of scapula.

T7: Inferior angle of scapula.

T12: Mid-point of vertical line between the inferior angle of the scapula and iliac crest.

L2: Renal arteries originate.

L4: Aorta bifurcates into the right and left common iliac arteries.

L4: Horizontal line between the highest point of the iliac crest.

S2: Sacral dimples mark the position of the posterior superior iliac spine are level with the S2.

Coccyx: Tip is palpable at the base of vertebral column between the gluteal masses.

Transpyloric Plane

- Body of L1
- Midway between jugular notch and pubic symphysis
- Duodenum
- Hila of kidneys
- Neck of pancreas
- Origin of superior mesenteric artery from aorta
- Celiac trunk
- Fundus of gallbladder.

Kidney: T12 to L3-4.

Spleen: Follows - rib10.

Pituitary fossa: Lies on the straight line joining the nasion with the inion at a depth of 6–7 cm from the nasion.

DR RATHI'S 17 IMPORTANT POINTS

1. X-rays were discovered by Wilhelm Conrad Roentgen in 1895.
2. Radioactivity was discovered by Henri Becquerel in 1896.
3. Radium was discovered by Marie and Pierre Curie in 1898.
4. One could achieve the same tumor response with less injury to normal tissue by fractionating the dose was proposed by Henri Coutard and Claude Regaud.
5. The Roentgen was internationally accepted as a unit of measurement for X-rays and gamma rays in 1928.
6. Rad as a unit of absorbed dose was recommended by the International Commission on Radiation Units (ICRU) in 1953.
7. The point of maximum electron equilibrium is referred to as D_{max}.
8. Percentage depth dose is dependent on field size, distance and energy.
9. The width of the penumbra increases with increased source-surface distance (SSD), decreased source-collimator distance, increased source size.
10. Required MeV is determined by multiplying the maximum tumor depth in centimeters by three.
11. The percentage depth dose at a given depth increases with higher beam energies.
12. The amount of back scatter increases with lower beam energies.
13. The most serious late consequence of high dose total body irradiation is radiation pneumonitis.
14. The exposure rate constant for radium is defined as the exposure rate at a point 1 cm away from 1 mg of radium filtered by 0.5 mm of platinum.
15. A beam spoiler is a sheet of lucite placed in the beam to reduce the depth of D_{max}.
16. To estimate the needed wedge angle in oblique fields subtract the hinge angle from 180 and divide by 2.
17. In an isocentric treatment technique, it is routine to normalize dose at isocenter.

CHAPTER 1

Basics of Radiation Therapy Planning

Gautam Saran

Radiotherapy is a clinical modality used in the treatment of primarily malignant tumors, and occasionally benign diseases, using electromagnetic and particulate radiations.

AIM OF RADIOTHERAPY

Delivering tumoricidal dose to a defined target volume, and respecting the normal tissue tolerance, thereby, trying to achieve an optimum therapeutic ratio.

STEPS IN RADIOTHERAPY PLANNING

Preplanning

- Evaluation and staging of tumor
- Intent of treatment
- Choice of treatment.

Planning Radiotherapy Treatment

- Treatment description
- Immobilization
- Simulation
- Image acquisition of tumor and patient data for planning
- Volume definition
- Choice of technique and beam modification
- Computation of dose distribution

Treatment Delivery

- Dose prescription
- Implementation of treatment
- Verification
- Monitoring treatment delivery and morbidity
- Recording and reporting.

Evaluation of Outcome

STEPS IN PREPLANNING

1. *Clinical evaluation and staging:*
   a. History and thorough clinical examination
   b. Confirmation of malignancy (cytology/histology)
   c. Appropriate investigations
      - To assess patient's general condition
      - Assess suitability to various treatment options
      - To know the local spread
      - Work-up of metastatic spread
      - Appropriate staging (TNM, FIGO, etc.).
2. *Intent of treatment:*
   a. *Radical:*
      - Intended to cure the patient of his or her disease
      - Area to be treated includes primary tumor and any other area having risk of disease
      - Radiation dose is higher hence some side effects are unavoidable, but these are acceptable as an inevitable part of attempted cure.
   b. *Palliative:*
      - To relieve distressing symptoms, e.g. hemoptysis, pain, bleeding, etc.
      - Simpler to execute and requires lesser treatment time
      - Comparatively lower dosage so as not to produce unacceptable side effects.

c. *Choice of treatment:*
- Ideally should be a tumor board decision
- Radiotherapy/surgery/chemotherapy/biotherapy or various combination
- If more than one treatment modality is required, then the sequences of these are decided.
  - *Primary treatment:* Definitive treatment
  - *Adjuvant treatment:* Treatment given in addition to definitive treatment
  - *Neoadjuvant (anterior) treatment:* Adjuvant treatment given prior to definitive treatment
  - *Concurrent treatment:* Two treatment modalities used together (e.g. concurrent [concomitant] chemoradiation as used in cervical cancer).

PLANNING RADIOTHERAPY TREATMENT

Description of Treatment

- Intent
- Choice of target volume
- Method of immobilization
- Treatment technique
- Machine and energy
- Dose prescription.

Patient Positioning and Immobilization

- Comfortable
- Reproducible
- Technically ideal
- Metallic prostheses, abdominal stomata, and pacemaker batteries must be identified and excluded from treatment field as much as possible.

- Immobilization and positioning devices
  - Neck rest
  - *Perspex shells and cast:* Head and neck, limbs
  - *Bite block:* Ensures constant chin extension and head immobilization
  - *Cork and tongue blade:* For positioning of tongue either in or out of treatment field
  - *Shoulder swing:* For lowering down the shoulder
  - *Window board:* Moving small bowel out of treatment field
  - *Breast board:* Treating breast cancer with tangential beams
  - *Vacuum bag:* For immobilization of any body part
  - *Brown-Robert-Wells (BRW) head ring and Gill-Thomas-Cosman (GTC) Relocatable head ring:* For stereotactic brain radiation.

Methods of Tumor Localization

- Tumor localization should be done exactly in the same position as subsequent treatments.
  - Identical patient positioning
  - Constant respiratory and urinary bladder filling
  - Identical couch specifications.
- Tumor data acquisition may involve
  - Clinical observations
  - Palpatory findings
  - Surgical details
  - Imaging (X-rays/USG/CT/MRI/PET/SPECT, etc.)
- Methods of target localization include
  - Simulator
  - CT scanning
  - Simulator-CT
  - CT-simulator

Simulator

The treatment simulator is essentially a specialized X-ray machine of diagnostic range which simulates all the movements and beam geometry of a radiotherapy treatment machine, viz.

- Beam divergence
- Beam direction
- SSD setting
- Field size
- Light beam shape.

It consists of:

- Isocentrically mounted X-ray machine, fluoroscopy set-up
- Couch capable to simulate treatment unit movements
- Gantry capable of rotating through 360 degrees
- Two pairs of crosswires mounted in the beam defining 50% isodose line.

Simulator-CT

- Essentially a simulator with a CT mode (of limited resolution) attached to the gantry
- Mainly used to obtain external contours though it may provide limited normal anatomical data helpful in inhomogeneity corrections
- Detailed tumor information is not obtained
- Less restriction on aperture size makes it suitable for planning larger fields, viz. breast, mantle technique, total body irradiation, etc.

CT-Simulator

- Essentially a CT scanner capable to generate images from beam's eye view.
- Image resolution is much better than a simulator-CT and hence detailed tumor information can be obtained.

- CT-simulator is better than simulator-CT in target volume delineation, dose calculation and simulation, where all can be done on one station.

Image Registration

- CT scan is ideal for planning
- It provides detailed density information for dose calculations of tissue inhomogeneity
- MRI and PETCT scan can be coregistered for more information.

Definition of Volumes

Gross Disease

- Macroscopic disease
- Can be seen/felt or detected by imaging
- Minimum number of cells is 10^9 (correlates to 1 cm in size and 1 gm in weight).

Microscopic Disease

- 10^6–10^9 number of cells
- Cannot be seen by naked eyes or imaging
- Detectable under microscope.

Subclinical Disease

- Less than 10^6 number of cells
- Cannot be seen even under microscope.

Dose required for disease control:

- *Subclinical disease:* 45–50 Gy
- *Microscopic disease:* 60–65 Gy
- *Gross disease:* 65–80 Gy.

ICRU 50 Report definitions:

a. *Gross tumor volume (GTV):*
   - Gross extent of malignant growth as determined by palpation or imaging study

- GTV primary—primary disease
- GTV nodal—involved nodes

b. *Clinical target volume (CTV):*
  - Tissue volume encompassing GTV and/or subclinical/microscopic disease
  - Natural avenues of spread, biological behavior of disease and micro extension must be taken into account while considering CTV.

  Both GTV and CTV are anatomical-clinical concepts.

c. *Planning target volume (PTV):*
  - It is static, geometric concept
  - Defined by specifying the margins that must be added around CTV to compensate the effects of:
    - Organ, tumor, and patient movements
    - Inaccuracies in beam and patient set-up.

d. *Treated volume:* Volume enclosed by an isodose surface that is selected and specified by radiation oncologists as being appropriate to achieve the purpose of treatment.

e. *Irradiated volume:* Volume that receives a dose considered significant in relation to normal tissue tolerance (e.g. 50% isodose surface).

f. *Organ at risk:* Normal tissue whose radiation sensitivity may significantly influence treatment planning or prescribed dose.

g. *ICRU reference point:*
  - Dose to the PTV be reported for the ICRU reference point, along with the minimum, maximum and mean dose.
  - ICRU reference point must be:
    - Defined in an unambiguous way
    - Clinically relevant
    - Located where the dose can be accurately determined
    - In a region in which, there are steep dose gradients, should be located at center of PTV and if possible of beam axes.

h. *Hot spot:* Volume >15 mm^3 in minimum diameter outside the PTV that receives >100% of the specified PTV dose (>105%).

i. *Cold spot:* The cold spot of target structure is defined as the ratio of the minimum dose received by any of the voxels of the structure to the prescription dose for that structure.

j. *Internal margin (IM):* It is situated around CTV or organ at risk and accounts for the uncertainties in anatomic information, physiologic changes such as expected movements and/or changes of shape and size of the CTV and RV in relation to reference points.

k. *Internal target volume (ITV):* It is defined by the outer boundary of the anatomically adjusted internal margin of the CTV.

l. *Internal risk volume (IRV):* It is defined by the outer boundary of the volume of organ at risk (RV).

Choice of Technique

a. *Treatment must be chosen according to:*
   - Percentage depth dose characterization and build up depth
   - Effect of penumbra or beam definition
   - Availability of independent or multileaf collimators
   - Facilities for both modification and portal imaging.

b. Dose specification point should be chosen according to ICRU recommendations. However, maximum and minimum target doses should be stated and the variation should ideally be limited to $\pm$ 5%.

c. *Dose specification points:*
   - Single beam—center of target volume
   - Two parallel opposed beams:
     - Equally weighted—mid plane point
     - Unequally weighted—center of target volume
   - Two or more intersecting beams—intersection of central axes
   - Rotation therapy (270°–360°)—center of rotation

- Rotation therapy with smaller axes—center of rotation, center of target volume.

d. *Choice of beam arrangement:*
   - Single direct beam
   - Parallel opposed beam
   - Combination of several beams.

e. *Beam modification devices:*
   - *Wedge filter (wedge):*
     - Wedge-shaped absorber which causes a progressive decrease in the intensity across the beam, resulting in a tilt of the isodose curves from their normal positions.
     - Usually made-up of lead or steel, it is mounted on transparent plastic tray which can be inserted in the beam at a specified distance from the source.
     - Wedge tray is kept at least 15 cm away from the skin surface, so as to avoid negating the skin—sparing effect of megavoltage beam
     - Wedge angle is the angle between the isodose curve and the normal to the central axis at a depth of 10 cm.
   - *Missing tissue compensator:*
     - It is needed to correct the dose inhomogeneity due to varying depth of target volume or obliquity of contours.
     - It can be bolus or compensatory filter.
     - Bolus is a tissue equivalent material (Lincolnshire bolus. 87% sugar and 13% magnesium carbonate, Spiers mixture 60% rice flour and 40% sodium bicarbonate) placed directly on the skin surface to even out the irregular contours of a patient to present a flat surface normal to the beam.
     - Build-up bolus is a bolus layer kept over skin surface (e.g. scar) to provide adequate dose build-up.
     - Placing bolus directly on the skin surface while using higher energy beams results in loss of skin sparing advantage.

– Instead, a compensating filter (usually made up of aluminum) may be used. It approximates the effect of bolus and preserves the skin sparing effect of megavoltage beam. Again, it is placed at a suitable (15–20 cm) from skin surface to avoid contamination with secondary electron.

- *Beam shaping block:*
  – They are used to shape the fields and reduce the amount of normal tissue irradiated.
  – Usually made up of a lead, they are placed on a tray attached to machine head. A thickness of four to five half value layers (HVL) is commonly used.
  – Multileaf collimators (MLCs) are another method (dynamic) of beam shaping.

Computation of Dose Distribution

- Percentage depth dose charts for varying field sizes and energy at fixed SSD are available for manual dose calculation.
- Instead, it can be done with the help of computerized program with beam data.

STEPS IN TREATMENT DELIVERY

Dose Prescription

- Total dose to the target volume
- Number of fractions
- Dose per fraction
- Overall treatment time
- Number of fractions per week
- Dose specification point.

Implementation, Verification and Monitoring of Treatment

- Patient is placed on the treatment couch exactly in the same manner as in the simulator, using all treatment aids.

- Patient is aligned using lasers.
- Beam parameters (size, gantry angle, wedges, compensators, collimator setting, etc.) are checked.
- SSD verified
- Ideally, clinician should monitor the first day treatment.
- *Verification can be done using:*
  - Port film
  - Electronic portal imaging, cone beam CT scan.

  Major limitations of port film are:
  - Delayed viewing due to processing time
  - It is impractical to do port films before each treatment
  - Poor quality images with megavoltage beams (especially > 6 MV) due to Compton effect.

Electron portal imaging (mirror based/liquid ion chamber based/solid state detector based) overcomes first two limitations of port film.

Table 1.1 Radiological factors controlling response to fractionated RT and their clinical relevance

Radiosensitivity	Intrinsic radiosensitivity differs between cells of tumors and normal tissue, and strongly determines final surviving fraction	Can account for variable response to tumors. Curative dose is proportional to the log of cell number
Repair	Cells differ in their capacity to repair DNA damage particularly after small dose of radiation usually more effective in nonproliferating cells The repair process takes at least 6 hours to complete	Repair is maximal in late responding tissue given small fractions Hyperfractionation may be advantageous Treatment should be well separated
Repopulation	Surrounding cells in many tumors and in acute responding normal tissue proliferate more rapidly once treatment is in progress	Accelerated therapy may be advantageous. Acute effect will be more
Reoxygenation	Hypoxic cells are radio-resistant. In between fraction; hypoxic cells re-oxygenate and become radiosensitive	Very short treatment time may lead to resistance due to persistence of hypoxic cells
Redistribution	Cells in 'S' phase are relatively radioresistant compared to that in G_2/M in between fractions; cells redistribute themselves over all phases of the cycle	Closely spaced treatment fractions may lead to resistance due to persistence of cells in less sensitive phase

Table 1.2 Causes of failure to control tumors by irradiation		
Tumor related	*Host related*	*Technical factors*
• Hypoxia	• Dose limiting normal tissues, e.g. tumor in close proximity to spinal cord	• Geographic miss
• Number of clonogenic cells	• Pathophysiologic factors, e.g. anemia in carcinoma cervix	• Calibration and calculation errors
• Growth and regeneration during treatment	• High immunogenic response	
• New primary tumor		
• Intrinsic radioresistance		
• Reseeding of irradiated areas		

Table 1.3 Calculation of gap junction
Methods of fields matching
• A 5–10 mm gap
• Use of half beam block
• Matching divergence of beams
• Use of moving junctions
• Simple matching of beams at the 50% margin defined by the light beam

CHAPTER 2

Head and Neck Cancer

Vikash Kumar, Ashutosh Mukherji

GENERAL PRINCIPLES AND OUTLINE OF MANAGEMENT

- History and clinical examination (local and systemic)
- Clinical staging
- Performance status and nutritional status
- Histopathology and cytology.

General Guidelines

- Stage I/II disease—single modality (surgery or radiotherapy)
- Stage III/IV disease—Surgery + Radiotherapy
  - Chemotherapy + Radiotherapy

Surgery preferred over radiotherapy (RT) as a single modality when:

- There is less morbidity after surgery
- Cosmesis and function are not a major concern
- Lesions involving or close to bone—to prevent radionecrosis
- Young patients.

Radiotherapy (RT) is preferred over surgery as a single modality when:

- High morbidity is expected after surgery
- Severe impairment of function and cosmesis can occur after surgery
- Surgery is difficult, i.e. radical excision is not possible
- Patient is unfit for surgery/refuses surgery.

Treatment Modalities

- Surgery—single modality in some early stage disease (I and II), along with radiotherapy in advanced disease, stage III and IV
- Radiotherapy—EBRT $\pm$ brachytherapy used in three different settings:
  - Radical curative radiotherapy $\pm$ chemotherapy
  - Postoperative adjuvant radiotherapy
  - Palliative radiotherapy

  3D CRT and IMRT are useful advances in RT techniques providing optimum therapeutic ratio.
- Chemotherapy—current evidence favors concurrent administration of chemoradiotherapy. In selected patients, chemotherapy has palliative role.

Treatment Intent

- Definitive or curative
- Palliative/supportive.

Definitive Treatment

- Stage I-IV A
- Prerequisites
  - Investigations
  - Dental review
  - Speech therapy/speech counseling
- Nutritional counseling and support.

Palliative/Supportive Care

- Stage IVB-IVC
- Poor general condition/performance status/advanced disease—needing counseling and supportive care
- Unresectable/metastatic disease with good general condition/performance status—needing chemotherapy with or without radiotherapy/altered fractionations.

PREREQUISITE INVESTIGATIONS FOR TREATMENT PLANNING

- X-ray chest PA view
- Ultrasound neck for N0 neck in selected cases
- OPG (orthopantomogram)/dental occlusion view
- EUA/endoscopy for tumor mapping
- CT scan/MRI for extent of disease
- Barium swallow
- PET-CT for evaluating recurrent/residual disease.

Reasons of Unresectability

Related to Primary

a. Base of skull involvement
b. Skin/soft tissue involvement
c. Infratemporal fossa involvement.

Related to Secondary

a. Infiltration to internal or common carotid artery
b. Clinically fixed node
c. Extensive infiltration of prevertebral muscle, skull base.

INDICATIONS FOR POSTOPERATIVE RADIOTHERAPY

Primary

- T3/T4 disease
- Close or positive margins of excision
- Deep infiltrative tumor
- Lymphovascular or perineural invasion.

Lymph Node

- Bulky nodal disease N2/N3
- Extranodal disease
- Multiple level involvement.

Decision to give postoperative radiation depends on:
- Stage of disease
- Spread pattern
- Excision margins status
- Perineural invasion
- Lymph node status including perinodal spread
- Differentiation.

Indications of Brachytherapy

- Site—oral cavity, base of tongue
- Localized disease (No disease)
- Small (T1) lesion
- Accessible site
- Substantial local recurrence rate
- Lesions away from bone.

Field Matching in Head and Neck Cancer Treatment

Conditions

- Matching orthogonal fields (parallel opposed and anterior)
- Matching photon and electron fields
- Positioning of lead shields.

Methods

- By calculating gap between the fields
- By using half beam block
- By matching beam divergence
- By using moving junction.

Patient Care

- Dental review
- Oral hygiene
- Cessation of smoking and alcohol

- Aspirin gargle
- Systemic analgesia
- Liquid/semisolid food
- High calorie food supplements
- Weekly weight/hematological assessment
- Nasogastric tubefeeding
- Tracheostomy in cases of ca larynx (airway compromised patients)
- Artificial saliva/artificial teardrop
- Shoulder physiotherapy
- Jaw stretching exercises to prevent postoperative trismus
- Swallowing and speech rehabilitation.

Radical Radiotherapy

1. Brachytherapy alone:
   T1-2 N0 – 60–70 Gy by LDR or equivalent by Ir^{192} HDR doses
2. Brachytherapy + EBRT:
   T1-3 N0-1 – EBRT – 56–60 Gy/28–30 fraction (#)/6 weeks
                     Boost brachytherapy – 15–20 Gy
3. EBRT alone:
   T1-4 N0-2 –   60–70 Gy/33–35 #/6–7 weeks (shrinking fields)
                 66–70 Gy/33–35#/6–7 weeks concurrent with CDDP 30 mg/m^2 weekly or 100 mg/m^2 3 weekly.

Postoperative Radiotherapy

Primary and nodal disease—50–60 Gy/25–30#/5–6 weeks using shrinking fields—site of residual disease, (+) margins—4–10 Gy boost.

Follow-up Protocol

- Every 2 months for first 2 years
- Six monthly for next 3 years
- Annually thereafter

- *Thorough clinical examination for:*
  - Locoregional control
  - Second primary
  - Late toxicities
  - T3, T4, TSH (neck irradiation).

ORAL CAVITY

Role of Radiotherapy

- *Buccal mucosa, floor of mouth, retromolar trigone:*
  - T1 and small T2 tumors are treated by radical implantation unless lesion extends close to bone/retromolar trigone
  - Larger lesions treated by a combination of external beam radiotherapy (EBRT) and implantation
  - In case of bone invasion; surgery followed by EBRT
  - In case of retromolar trigone, surgery followed by post-operative EBRT or EBRT alone as these sites are difficult to approach for implant
- *Tongue:*
  - Surgery for small superficial tumors
  - Interstitial implants for T1 and small T2 tumors
  - External beam radiotherapy followed by interstitial implantation for larger T2 and T3 lesion
  - Early tumors with mobile lymph nodes—surgery/interstitial implant for primary and neck dissection for lymph nodes.

Planning Technique

Disease Assessment

- Clinical
- Evaluation under anesthesia for tumor mapping
- Radiological—Orthopantomogram, CECT, MRI, PET scan

Simulation

- Supine position with Perspex cast
- Mouthbite
- Straight neck
- Demarcation of palpable nodes with wire

Buccal Mucosa

- *Brachytherapy:* Single plane/double plane implant according to tumor thickness.
- *EBRT:*
    - Target volume for buccal mucosa—primary tumor + 2 cm margin + ipsilateral submandibular lymph node.

    Field arrangement: Small anterior and ipsilateral-wedged fields in case of unilateral disease (**Fig. 2.1**).

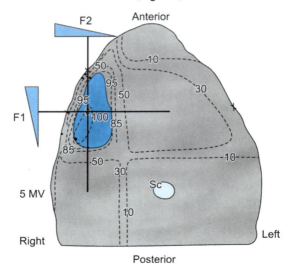

Fig. 2.1 Typical field arrangement for radiation therapy of small tumor of the buccal mucosa, F1: Gantry 270°, 45° wedge, weight 100%, 5.5 × 7 cm, F2: Gantry 0°, 45° wedge, weight 120%, 4 × 7 cm

– *Target volume for lower alveolus:* Mandible on affected side plus submental and submandibular lymph node.

Field arrangement: Oblique anterior and lateral-wedged field **(Fig. 2.2).**

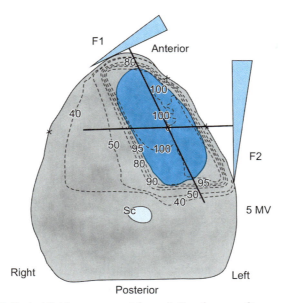

Fig. 2.2 Typical field arrangement for radiation therapy of tumor of the lower alveolus, F1: Gantry 335°, 45° wedge, weight 85%, 5.5 × 6.5 cm, F2: Gantry 90°, 30° wedge, weight 100%, 8.5 × 6.5 cm

Lip

T1, T2	– Sx (wide excision)
	RT (radical radiotherapy/brachytherapy)
T3, T4	– Sx + postoperative radiotherapy
N_0	– Observe or SOHD
N^+	– MND (modified neck dissection).

Tongue

Brachytherapy

- *Tumor <1 cm:* Hairpin technique
- *Tumor upto 2 cm:* Plastic loop technique.

External Beam Radiotherapy (EBRT)

T2 diseases which are unsuitable for surgery plus EBRT and implantation treated by external radiotherapy; target volume includes tumor plus 2 cm margin and ipsilateral submandibular and deep cervical lymph nodes (**Fig. 2.3**).
Field arrangement: Anterior and lateral-wedged fields.
Large T2 and T3 disease spread is across midline.
Field arrangement: Parallel opposed lateral fields are used.

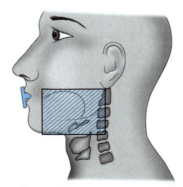

Fig. 2.3 Margins of lateral field for localized carcinoma of the tongue

Floor of Mouth

Brachytherapy techniques are similar to those of tongue.

EBRT

T1 and small T2 disease:
Field arrangement: Two anterior oblique wedged fields are used **(Fig. 2.4)**.

T2–T4 disease:
Field arrangement: Two parallel opposed lateral fields are used.

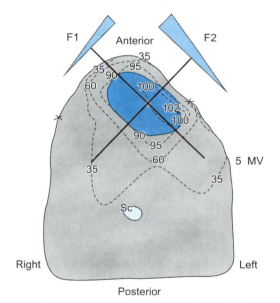

Fig. 2.4 Typical isodose for anterior-wedged oblique fields to treat small anterior floor of mouth tumor. F1: Gantry 315°, 30° wedge, weight 120%, 5 × 6 cm; F2: Gantry 45°, 40° wedge, weight 100%, 6.5 × 6 cm

Retromolar Trigone

Site is unsuitable for brachytherapy.

EBRT

T1, T2 disease—anterior and posterior oblique-wedged fields are used. If there is palpable lymph node; neck is treated with separate anterior field.

T3 and T4 disease—two parallel opposed fields are used. Neck is treated with separate anterior field.

Lower alveolus and retromolar trigone:
- *Mandible uninvolved:*
  - Surgery – wide excision with marginal mandibulectomy ± SOHD for N0 disease MND for N+ disease
  - Postoperative radiotherapy is indicated as per earlier guidelines.
- *Mandible grossly involved:*
  - Surgery + adjuvant radiotherapy
  - Surgery – wide excision and segmental/hemi-mandibulectomy + SOHD for N0 and MND/RND for N+ disease
  - Postoperative radiotherapy as per earlier guidelines.

Dose

Brachytherapy

- *Radical treatment:* 65–70 Gy to the 85% reference isodose using Paris system.
- *Boost treatment:* 25–30 Gy to the 85% reference isodose using Paris system.

EBRT

Radical treatment: 66–70 Gy in 33–35 fractions over 6.5–7 weeks.
Preimplantation: 40–50 Gy in 20–25 fractions given in 4–5 weeks.

MAXILLARY ANTRUM

Infrastructure and suprastructure disease divided by Ohngren's line.

Criteria for Unresectability
- Gross infiltration of infratemporal fossa
- Pterygopalatine fissure involvement
- Involvement of dura and intracerebral extensions
- Cavernous sinus involvement
- Involvement of sphenoid
- Extensive soft tissue and skin infiltration
- Bilateral orbital involvement.

Role of Radiotherapy

For T1 and T2 disease of infrastructure partial maxillectomy alone can lead to high control rate.

For advanced disease; total maxillectomy and radiotherapy is treatment of choice.

Definitive radiotherapy is indicated in:
- Medically unfit patients
- Those who refuse surgery
- Extensive inoperable disease.

Planning Technique

Assessment of primary disease by:
- Local examination
- X-ray PNS
- CECT.

In case maxillectomy has not been performed; drainage by intranasal antrostomy/Caldwell-Luc procedure is advised.

Target Volume

a. *Anterior field:*
   - *Upper border:* Supraorbital ridge
   - *Lower border:* Hard palate
   - *Medial border:* Contralateral inner canthus

- *Lateral border:* Gingivobuccal sulcus
- *Anterior border:* Cheek.
b. *Lateral field:*
  - *Anterior border:* Just behind the lateral bony margin of the orbit
  - *Posterior border:* Just before tragus
  - Upper and lower border correspond to the anterior field.

Field Arrangements *(Fig. 2.5)*

- Anterior and lateral wedged fields are used.
- Lateral field is angled 5–10° posteriorly.
- If posteromedial part is involved, then an additional contralateral wedged field is used.
- Hypothalalmus and optic chiasm are shielded in lateral field.
- If orbit is spared, then cornea, lens and lacrimal apparatus are shielded in anterior field.

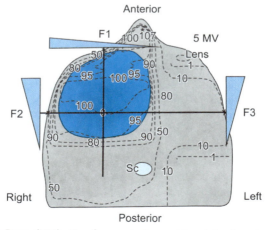

Fig. 2.5 Dose distribution from anterior and two lateral wedged fields with differential weighing. F1: Gantry 10°, 15° wedge, weight 100%, 9 × 8 cm; F2: Gantry 270°, 60° wedge, weight 15%, 6 × 8 cm; F3: Gantry 90°, 60° wedge, weight 15%, 6 × 8 cm

- If orbit is involved; cornea is protected by cutting out cast, treating with eye open and the patient is asked to look into the beam.
- If cheek or anterior nasal cavity is involved; anterior field is kept open.

Dose Suggested

T_1/T_2: 66 Gy in 33 fractions given in 6.5 weeks for radical RT.
T_3/T_4: 70 GY/ 35 fractions in 7 weeks.

Nasal Cavity and Ethmoid Sinuses

- *Limited disease:* Target volume—It includes medial maxillary sinus, ethmoid sinus, medial portion of orbit, nasopharynx, sphenoid sinus and base of skull.
- Advanced disease and ethmoid sinus tumors are managed in similar fashions.
- Treatment is heavily weighted towards the anterior field (8:1 or 10:1 in favor of anterior field).
- To boost the primary; open anterior field is used to concentrate dose to major bulk of disease.
- If orbit is involved minimally, the major lacrimal gland and lateral upper eyelid is shielded.
- If most of the orbit is involved; entire orbital content is included in the field.

NASOPHARYNX

Role of Radiotherapy

- For all stages; radiotherapy is treatment of choice and intent is radical.
- Bilateral neck irradiation is mandatory even if the involvement is unilateral.
- T3, T4 disease with any N status, concurrent chemotherapy and radiotherapy is preferred over radiotherapy alone.

Planning Technique

Assessment of Disease

- Rhinoscopy
- Examination of pharynx and larynx for tumor extension and cranial nerve involvement
- Examination of cranial nerve and cervical sympathetic chain
- Examination of ear for Eustachian tube obstruction
- Lateral X-rays of neck including skull base and petrous bone
- CECT.

Target Volume

Comprises primary tumor, entire lymphatic system and the potential routes of spread. It includes—

- Base of skull
- Floor of middle cranial fossa
- Posterior half of nasal cavity and orbit
- Sphenoid and posterior ethmoid sinuses
- Parapharyngeal space
- Lymph nodes lateral pharyngeal, posterior cervical, deep cervical and supraclavicular lymph node.

Simulation

- Supine with neck extended but keeping the spinal cord straight.
- Lateral orbital margins and nodes are marked with wire.

Field Arrangements *(Fig. 2.6)*

a. *Patients without lymphadenopathy:*
  - Parallel opposed lateral fields for primary disease with a separate anterior neck field for cervical lymph node is used.
  - To boost primary; fields are shrinked to gross disease and a two lateral wedged and one anterior field is used.

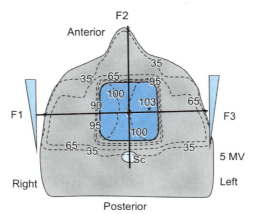

Fig. 2.6 Dose distribution from an anterior and two lateral fields. F1: Gantry 270° 30° wedge, weight 100% 7 × 8 cm, F2: Gantry 0°, weight 100% 6.5 × 8 cm, F3: Gantry 90° 30° wedge, weight 100% 7 × 8 cm

b. *Patients with lymphadenopathy:*
   • Parallel opposed lateral fields covering the entire target volume including the spinal cord.
   • Anterior half of orbit, optic chiasm, part of brainstem is shielded.
   • Lower half of the neck including supraclavicular is treated with separate anterior field and care should be taken in defining the junction that it should not overlie the palpable disease.
   • If there is involvement of anterior nasal cavity; an additional anterior field is used. Anterior and lateral fields are treated isocentrically.
   • Central shielding is used to protect larynx and spinal cord.

Dose Suggested

a. *Patients without lymphadenopathy:*
   • Nasopharyngeal and neck fields—56 Gy in 28 fractions given in 5.5 weeks.

- Nasopharynx alone—10–14 Gy in 5–8 fractions in 1–1.5 weeks.
b. *Patients with lymphadenopathy:*
  - Large lateral fields 40 Gy in 20 fractions over 4 weeks.
  - Nasopharyngeal fields (boost) 26 Gy in 13 fractions over 2.5 weeks.
  - Neck field boost 26 Gy in 13 fractions over 2.5 weeks.

OROPHARYNX

Role of Radiotherapy

- Early T1-T2 tumors treated best by radiotherapy alone as surgery leads to severe morbidities.
- T3-T4 diseases are best treated by concomitant chemotherapy + radiotherapy. Surgery is added if low perioperative risk and reasonable functional outcome.
- T1-T2, N2-N3 concomitant CT + radiotherapy in most cases followed by Neck salvage if residual nodes are present.
- Sixty percent of patients present with lymphadenopathy, however, even in node negative patients elective neck irradiation is done.
- Mobile unilateral nodes are best treated by block dissection followed by radiotherapy.
- Fixed bilateral nodes are treated by radical radiotherapy; surgery if residual nodes are there.

Planning Technique

Assessment of Disease

- Clinical assessment
- Indirect/direct laryngoscopy
- X-ray soft tissue neck
- CECT.

Target Volume

- *Upper border:* Hard palate
- *Lower border:* Clavicle
- *Anterior margin:* Anterior border of masseter
- *Posterior margin:* Vertical line from tip of mastoid or is further extended posteriorly to include bulky cervical lymph node
- *Medial margin:* Midline.

Simulation

- Supine with straight neck, no mouth bite.
- Wires to outline lymph nodes.

Field Arrangements

- *Wedged pair technique:* Anterior and posterior oblique wedged fields for small primary tumors.
- *Opposing lateral fields:* For larger primary; parallel opposed lateral fields are used.

In some situations like in tonsillar tumors 2:1 weighting is required to give high dose to the primary and ipsilateral lymph nodes and prophylactic irradiation to contralateral tonsil and deep cervical lymph nodes.

In case, if tongue base or soft palate is involved equal weightage is used for adequate dose to the both primary and lymph nodes.

If there is involvement of upper deep cervical lymph nodes; the neck below the opposing lateral fields is treated using an anterior field with shielding to larynx and spinal cord.

Dose Prescription

- 66 Gy in 33 fractions over 6.5 weeks for $T_1 - T_2$ (nonbulky).
- 70 Gy in 35 fractions over 7 weeks for T_2 (bulky) $- T_4$.

LARYNX

Choice of treatment depends upon:
- Voice preservation
- Local control rate
- Fitness for surgery
- Reliability of follow-up.

Role of Radiotherapy

Glottic Tumors

- T1 and T2 diseases are best treated with radical radiotherapy.
- 5-year survival rates 80–95%.
- Local recurrence rate is 10–20% for T1 disease and 25–30% for T2 disease.
- T3 diseases have comparable results with radiotherapy and surgery; 5-year survival rate being 50%.

Supraglottic Tumors

- T1 and T2 supraglottic tumors are treated by radiotherapy or partial laryngectomy.
- T3 and T4 lesions are treated by laryngectomy and postoperative radiotherapy.

Subglottic Tumors

- T1 and T2 supraglottic tumors are treated by radiotherapy or partial laryngectomy.
- T3 and T4 lesions are treated by laryngectomy and postoperative radiotherapy.

Planning Technique

Assessment of Disease

- Palpation for laryngeal crepitus and cervical lymph nodes
- Indirect and direct laryngoscopy

- Chest X-ray
- X-ray soft tissue neck
- Barium swallow
- CT scan, MRI.

Give information regarding:
- Extent of disease
- Cartilage invasion
- Extralaryngeal spread
- Para/Pre-epiglottic space invasion
- Nodal status.

Target Volume

Glottic tumors:
- T1-T2 disease—5 × 5 field size is taken, center of which lies at 1 cm below the promontory of thyroid cartilage. If T2 disease is associated with supraglottic or subglottic extension; volume is larger to include the extensions and margins.
- For T3 and T4 disease radiotherapy is used in postoperative setting and target volume is individualized to cover the potential sites of recurrence.

Supraglottic tumors: For N0 disease; target volume includes primary tumor, upper deep cervical and midjugular lymph nodes. *Upper margin* includes tonsillar margin. *Posterior margin* is a vertical line from the tip of mastoid process. Inferior margin is extended up to clavicle.

Boost volume encompasses primary tumor alone.

For patients with palpable cervical lymph nodes; target volume includes primary tumor with bilateral deep cervical chain and supraclavicular lymph nodes.

Subglottic tumors: Target volume is primary tumor, pre- and paratracheal lymph nodes, lower jugular lymph nodes and superior mediastinum.

Simulation

Patient is treated in supine position with straight neck. Palpable lymph nodes are marked with wire. Target volume and spinal cord are simulated in both lateral and AP views.

Field Arrangements

Glottic: Two parallel opposed lateral wedged (15° or 30°) portal is used to compensate for changing contours in neck **(Fig. 2.7)**.

Special cases
- *Obese patients:* Two anterior oblique wedged portals are used to spare skin in lateral side of neck. To avoid spinal cord; gantry angle is chosen 45°–60° **(Fig. 2.8)**.

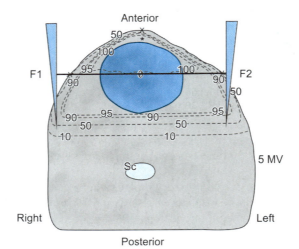

Fig. 2.7 Two opposing lateral wedged fields for treatment of a T1 glottic tumor. F1: Gantry 270° 15° wedge, weight 100% 5 × 5 cm, F2: Gantry 90° 15° wedge, weight 100% 5 × 5 cm

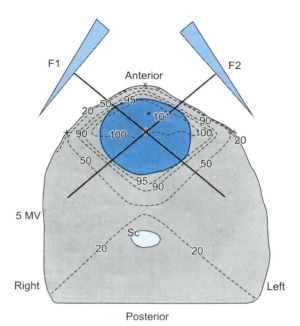

Fig. 2.8 Two anterior oblique fields for treatment of early glottic carcinoma. F1: Gantry 310°, 30° wedge, weight 100%, 5 × 6 cm; F2: Gantry 50°, 30° wedge, weight 100%, 5 × 5 cm

- *Anterior commissure involvement:* Two parallel opposed lateral portals with bolus in front of the larynx or two parallel opposed lateral wedged (15°) portal is used.
- Advanced disease are treated using parallel opposed lateral portal.

Supraglottic: For N0 disease; parallel opposed lateral wedged (15°) portal with equal weightage is used.

For N+ disease the primary site and upper and middle cervical lymph nodes are treated using parallel opposed lateral fields while the lower cervical lymph nodes and supraclavicular lymph nodes are treated by matched anterior fields. Boost is delivered by parallel opposed fields to primary disease and nodes sparing the spinal cord. If there is massive cervical lymphadenopathy overlying the spinal cord; boost is delivered using electron beam with suitable energy.

Subglottic: Two parallel opposed lateral wedged fields angled inferiorly and an anterior field with longitudinal wedge covering up to superior mediastinum is used.

- Lung apices are shielded with lead blocks.
- Lateral fields are angled inferiorly by using couch twist of 30°.

Boost is delivered by parallel opposed fields to primary disease and nodes sparing the spinal cord. If there is cervical nodes overlying the spinal cord; boost is delivered using electron beam with suitable energy.

Dose

- 66 Gy in 33 fractions over 6.5 weeks.
- In postoperative settings, 58–60 Gy is required.

Hypopharynx

Role of Radiotherapy

For pyriform fossa; radiotherapy is used in postoperative settings to reduce the local recurrence as these tumors present with advanced disease.

Indications of radical radiotherapy:
- Early medial wall tumors
- Patients unfit for surgery
- Palliative settings in T4, N3 disease.

For postcricoid tumors without lymphadenopathy or with mobile lymph node; TOC is laryngopharyngectomy. Radical RT is given in palliative settings for advanced cases.

For posterior pharyngeal wall tumors; radical radiotherapy is treatment of choice.

Assessment of Disease

- Indirect and direct laryngoscopy
- Chest X-ray
- X-ray soft tissue neck
- Barium swallow
- CT scan, MRI.

Target Volume

Pyriform fossa (T1/T2 disease with N0 or minimal lymphadenopathy)
- Upper margin—angle of mouth
- Lower margin—lower border of cricoid cartilage
- Posterior border lies in front of spinal cord.

Boost volume includes primary tumor and grossly involved lymph node.

Parallel opposed lateral portal is used.

Patient is treated in supine cast and asked to keep the neck straight.

Dose:
- Initial target volume—50 Gy in 25 fractions over 5 weeks
- Boost—16 Gy in 8 fractions over 10 days.

Pyriform fossa (T3 disease with extensive lymphadenopathy)
- Upper margin—angle of mouth
- Lower margin—up to clavicle
- Posterior margin is individualized to include the cervical lymph nodes
- Boost volume includes primary tumor and grossly involved lymph node
- Parallel opposed lateral portal is used

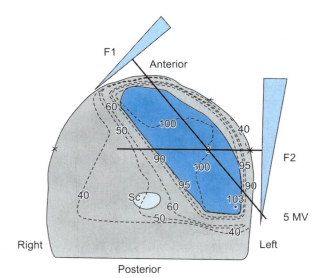

Fig. 2.9 Isodose distribution for treatment of T3 pyriform fossa tumor with node mass. F1: Gantry 320° 30° wedge, weight 90% 6 × 9 cm, F2: Gantry 90° 30° wedge, weight 100% 9 × 9 cm

- Patient is treated in supine cast with chin extended to displace oral cavity and mandible out of treatment field.

  If lymph nodes are overlying the spinal cord; the dose beyond the cord tolerance is delivered by either electron boost or a wedged lateral field and a contralateral anterior oblique field **(Fig. 2.9)**.

Dose
66 Gy in 33 fractions over 6.5 weeks.

Postcricoid Region

Radical radiotherapy: Indicated in patients without lymph nodal involvement. T1 and T2—Radical RT, T3 and T4—CT-RT.

- Target volume includes primary disease including inferior spread into the cervical esophagus and adjacent lymphatics.

- Patient is treated in a supine cast keeping the neck straight.
- Two lateral wedged (10°) portals angled inferiorly with equal weightage is used to increase dose to superior mediastinum and cervical esophagus.
- Gantry angle, couch angle and head twist are adjusted to achieve desired dose distribution.

Dose
66 Gy in 33 fractions over 6.5 weeks.

Posterior Pharyngeal Wall

Target volume: Whole hypopharynx, bilateral deep cervical lymph nodes and retropharyngeal space with 2 cm margins.

Patient is asked to keep the neck straight.

Parallel opposed wedged (15°) lateral portal is used.

If there is extension to cervical esophagus, the beam is angulated inferiorly.

Dose
66 Gy in 33 fractions over 6.5 weeks.

Parotid Tumors

Surgical Options

- Superficial parotidectomy
- *Total parotidectomy in cases with:*
  - Deep lobe tumors
  - High grade tumors
  - Positive margins following superficial parotidectomy
- *Radical parotidectomy when involving:*
  - Skin
  - Infratemporal fossa
  - Mandible
  - Petrous bone.

Role of Radiotherapy

- *Benign tumors:*
  - Inadequate surgery
  - Tumor spillage
  - Recurrence
- *Malignant tumors:*
  - Positive or very close margins
  - High-grade histology
  - Positive nodes
  - Extensive perineural spread
  - Skin or bone involvement
  - Recurrence
  - Palliation
  - T3/T4 disease
  - Adenoid cystic carcinoma
  - Deep lobe tumors.

Assessment of Disease

Clinical: For
- Facial nerve involvement
- Trismus
- Associated lymphadenopathy.

Radiological: CECT.

Target Volume

- *Upper margin:* 1 cm above the zygomatic arch
- *Lower margin:* 1 cm below the angle of mandible
- *Anterior margin:* Anterior border of masseter
- *Posterior margin:* Mastoid process
- *Lateral margin:* Includes the scar/palpable disease
- *Medial margin:* Covers the parapharyngeal space.

Special Cases

Adenoid cystic carcinoma:
- Perineural spread
- Target volume is extended superiorly up to base of skull and entire facial nerve up to petrous temporal bone.

Undifferentiated or squamous cell carcinoma: Entire ipsilateral lymphatic drainage of neck is treated.

Simulation:
- Patient lies supine and neck extended to make superior margin perpendicular to the couch top.
- No mouth bite is needed.
- Operative scars and palpable disease is marked with radiopaque wire.

Beam arrangement:
- Anterior and posterior oblique wedged (45°) portals with equal weightage **(Fig. 2.10)**.
- If patient is unable to extend his neck, or if target volume needs to include base of skull, the plane of posterior beam is inclined downwards by 10–15°.

Dose prescription:
- Macroscopic disease—66 Gy in 33 # over 6.5 weeks.
- Microscopic disease—60 Gy in 30 # over 6 weeks.
- Benign disease—55 Gy in 27 # over 5.5 weeks.

EAR

Role of Radiotherapy
- Usually given in postoperative settings
- Palliative settings
- Inoperable cases.

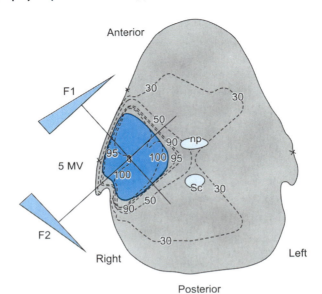

Fig. 2.10 Anterior and posterior oblique wedged fields for treatment of a parotid tumor; F1: Gantry 320° 45° wedge, weight 100% 7.5 × 8 cm, F2: Gantry 230° 45° wedge, weight 100% 7 × 8 cm

Assessment of Disease

- Clinical examination
  - Parotid region
  - Ear
  - Facial nerve
  - Mastoid region
  - Regional lymphatics
- Otoscopy
- CT scan.

Target Volume

It is triangular volume with apex towards brainstem.
- *Upper border:* Inferior orbital margin
- *Lower border:* Tip of mastoid
- *Anterior border:* Covers the preauricular and parotid lymph nodes
- *Posterior border:* Includes postauricular lymph nodes.

Simulation

Supine and neck extended to make superior margin to cross at upper border of pinna and to keep treatment plane perpendicular to table top.

Beam Arrangements

- Anterior and posterior oblique-wedged (45°) portals with equal weightage is used.
- Posterior portal is aligned so that the beam exits below the contralateral eye.

Dose

66 Gy in 33 # over 6.5 weeks.

Unknown Primary

Treatment depends upon:
- The location of lymph nodes.
- Histology.
- If upper and middle jugular lymph nodal involvement is present, elective irradiation of the nasopharynx, oropharynx, supraglottic larynx and hypopharynx is done via parallel opposed portal, lower neck, up to the level of clavicle is treated by separated anterior field.

- If a primary focus is suspected but has no proof, an extra boost dose may be added to this specific site.
- A node in the upper neck with histologic findings suggestive of lymphoepithelioma, elective irradiation of nasopharynx and oropharynx is done.
- A solitary lymph node in submandibular region is involved, then treatment is neck dissection with observation because irradiation to entire oral cavity with neck causes severe morbidities.
- A preauricular lymph node with SCC histology represents mets from a skin cancer and is treated by combination of parotidectomy and radiation therapy or RT alone.
- Supraclavicular lymph node treated with generous regional portal which includes adjacent apex of axilla.

MINOR SALIVARY GLAND TUMORS

- Surgery is the treatment of choice for both benign and malignant tumors (wide excision is preferred).
- Radiation therapy significantly decreases locoregional recurrence rate.
- Technique of radiation is similar to that of squamous cell carcinoma at the corresponding primary site.
- For postoperative RT 6000–6500 cGy over 6–7 weeks is given.
- For early stage disease 7000–7500 cGy over 7–7.5 weeks is used.

UNUSUAL NONEPITHELIAL TUMORS

Glomus Tumor (Chemodectomas/Paragangliomas)

- Common sites in head and neck region:
  - Middle ear—glomus tympanicum
  - Carotid body—glomus jugulare
  - Others—orbit, larynx, nasal, etc.
- Usually benign in nature, although can metastasize or be locally malignant.

- *Treatment:*
  - Surgery for smaller tumors and those which are less likely to be associated with significant operative morbidity
  - Indications for RT:
    - Larger tumors
    - Inoperable sites: glomus jugulare, glomus tympanicum
    - Extensive bone destruction
    - Intracranial involvement
    - Jugular foramen syndrome
    - Usually two parallel opposed portal is used for relatively localized glomus tumors
    - Dose–45–55 Gy in 5 weeks
    - For glomus tympanicum; three field arrangement with superior-inferior wedged (60° and 45°) and open lateral field is used with weightage 1:1 : 0.33.
- *Other options are:*
  - Electron beam with a lateral portal
  - Electron + proton (80% + 20%) combination
  - Stereotactic radiosurgery (SRS) and 3D-CRT.

Hemangiopericytomas

- Role of radiotherapy—mainly in adjuvant setting after complete excision or after minimal residual disease
- In head and neck regions; nasal cavity and orbit are the usual location
- Field of irradiation should be wide to encompass the tumor with at least 5 cm margin to encompass the tumor bed
- *Dose:* 60–65 Gy in 6–7 weeks.

Chordomas

- In head and neck region, clivus is the usual site
- Radiation therapy is indicated in postoperative settings

- Field arrangement—parallel opposed lateral wedged portal with an open anterior field
- Depending upon the position combination of photon and electron beams are used
- *Dose:* 50 Gy in 25 # over 5 weeks.

Lethal Midline Granulomas

- Most patients have involvement of the nasal cavity and PNS, however, the lesion may extend to the orbits, palate and pharynx
- Target volume should include all areas of involvement including adjacent areas at risk with a generous 2–3 cm margin
- Field and portal depend upon the site of involvement and extent
- *Dose prescription:* 45–50 Gy in 4.5–5.5 weeks.

Chloromas

- Usually along with AML (M4/M5)
- Most commonly found in association with bone and nervous tissues
- The most common sites of presentation are orbit and other craniofacial bones
- Extremely radiosensitive
- Technique depends upon the location of the infiltrate
- *Dose:* 30 Gy in 15 # over 3 weeks
- Superficial lesions—electron beam is recommended

Esthesioneuroblastoma

- Indications of radiotherapy (postoperative)
  - High grade tumor
  - Locally advanced disease
- Early lesions with little or no bony destructions or nerve invasions can be treated adequately with radical RT.

Radiation Therapy Techniques

- For anteriorly situated tumors combination of photon and electron beams is preferred
- For intracranial/posteriorly situated tumors; or in case if there is maxillary extension a pair of perpendicular anteroposterior and lateral wedged portal or two lateral wedged and an open anterior portal is used
- In postoperative cases, tissue defects are compensated by bolus/obturator
- Neck irradiation is indicated in Kadish stage with disease (44% chance in stage C, 10% in stage A/B).

Dose Prescription

- Postoperative setting – 50–60 Gy in 25 – 30 # over 5–6 weeks
- Radical dose – 65–70 Gy in 32–35 # over 6.5–7 weeks.

Extramedullary Plasmacytomas

- Constitutes 0.5% of all upper respiratory tract malignancies
- Most common sites are the nasopharynx, nasal cavity, para-nasal sinuses and tonsils
- Surgery is advised for pedunculated lesions; for all other lesions TOC is radiation therapy (local control rate 85%)
- Techniques of irradiation depends upon the location of primary tumors
- *Dose prescription:* 50–60 Gy in 25–30 Gy over 5–6 weeks.

Juvenile Nasopharyngeal Angiofibroma

- 0.05% of head and neck tumors
- For extracranial tumors; surgery is TOC
- *Radiation therapy is indicated in:*
  - Tumors with intracranial extensions
  - Recurrent tumors

- *Radiation therapy techniques:*
  - Treatment portals resemble those of nasopharynx with irradiation of cervical lymph node
  - If there is extension into the nasal cavity/PNS treatment portals resemble to those of PNS
  - Usually two parallel opposed lateral portal of size 6 × 6 or 8 × 8 cm with compensators for inhomogeneity correction in nasal area
  - More extensive disease requires three-field wedge pair techniques
- *Dose prescription:* 30 – 50 Gy in 15–25 #.

GLOMUS JUGULARE

Indications for Radiotherapy

- Preoperatively or postoperatively
- Postsurgery recurrence
- Tumors with destruction of petrous bone, jugular fossa, occipital bone
- Patients with jugular foramen syndrome (paralysis of cranial nerves IX – XI).

Dose of Radiotherapy

Total dose of 45–55 Gy in 5 weeks for benign glomus tumors and 65–70 Gy in 6.5 weeks for malignant glomus tumors to the PTV @180–200 cGy per fraction 5 times a week is generally sufficient in more than 80% cases for local control.

Volume and Technique of Radiotherapy

- Limited bilateral wedged portals used. Three field technique may be used in larger tumors. In case of extension to posterior fossa, parallel opposed portals are used.

- 3D-CRT or IMRT may be considered for better dose distribution.
- 15–18 MeV electrons used alone or in combination with 4–6 MV photons are used (photons for 20–25% of total tumor dose). In case of posterior fossa spread, 6–18 MV photons used.
- 45- or 60-degree wedged fields used.

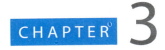

Gynecologic Tumors

Kanika Sharma

UTERINE CANCER

Role of Radiotherapy

Medically inoperable stage I and II disease.
Adjuvant in Stage I_A G_3, I_B G_3.
Stage II and III (when surgery reveals high-risk factors such as adnexal or parametrial involvement, cervical stromal involvement, pelvic nodal involvement, high tumor grade, papillary/serous cell type, lymphovascular space invasion, invasion of myometrium to more than half its thickness).

Assessment of Primary Tumor

- Clinical assessment and local examination
- EUA-biopsy and fractional curettage from uterus MRI scan.

Target Delineation

- Target volume—primary up to upper 2/3 vagina, and entire vagina in clear cell variants
- Pelvic nodes (internal/external/common iliac).

Radiotherapy Technique

Patient positioning: Supine.
Portals: Anteroposterior opposing or four field technique.

Field Placements Borders

- *Superior:* L_4/L_5 interspace
- *Inferior:* Mid-obturator foramen
- *Lateral:* 1.5–2 cm from widest true pelvis.

Alternatively, four-field technique by adding lateral portals for which borders are:

- Anterior margin—symphysis pubis
- Posterior margin—covers 50% of rectum in I_B
- Sacral hollow S_2—S_3 interspace in advanced disease
- Superior margin—inferior edge of L_4
- Inferior margin—inferior edge of ischium.
- *Beam energy:*
  - Use four fields when using telecobalt or 4–6 MV X-rays
  - 15–18 MV X-ray.

DOSE PRESCRIPTION

Preoperative

45 Gy/25 fraction/5weeks@1.8 Gy/# followed by brachy therapy application 7 Gy × 3 fractions by HDR. Alternatively 9 Gy × 2 fractions by HDR.

Postoperative

- 50 Gy/25#/5 weeks @ 2 Gy/# treating 5 days a week
- ICRT with vaginal applicators
- LDR-30 Gy at 0.5 cm from the applicator surface, treating upper 2/3rd of vagina
- HDR-2# of 5.5 Gy or 6 Gy/3# at 0.5 cm from the applicator surface
- If vaginal cuff RT alone, then 6 Gy × 5 or 6 (HDR) or 60–70 Gy (LDR) to vaginal surface.

Patient Care

Skin reaction in sacral and perineal regions is common. Exposure to air and keeping skin dry. One percent hydrocortisone cream reduces erythema and irritation. Low residue diet. Diarrhea is treated when necessary. If severe, interrupt treatment or reduce dose per fraction.

CARCINOMA CERVIX

Role of Radiation Therapy

- Stage I_B II_A selected cases
- Stage II_B onwards—for bulky disease with subsequent ICRT.

Assessment of Primary Tumor

- Clinical assessment with local examination for the extent of disease (P/S, P/V, P/R).

EUA: Four quadrant biopsy and fractional curettage from uterus Cystoscopy, IVP, MRI.

Target Delineation

Target Volume

Primary tumor and pelvic nodes (Pelvic nodes [internal/external/common iliac).

Radiotherapy Technique

Patient Positioning—Supine

- Parallel opposing fields or four-field technique
- Size of portal depends on the extent of disease.

Field Placement Borders

- *Superior:* L_4/L_5 interspace (if common iliac nodes, then L_3/L_4 interspace)

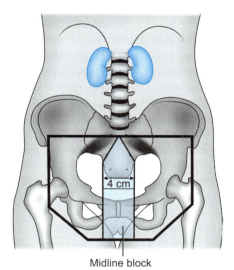

Midline block

Fig. 3.1 Radiation fields for inguinal and pelvic nodal irradiation

- *Inferior:*
  - Inferior obturator foramen, if no vaginal involvement
  - Entire vagina, if vaginal extension present in lower 1/3rd
  - Inguinal LN included if distal vagina involved **(Fig. 3.1)**
- *Lateral:* 1.5–2 cm from widest true pelvis
- *Alternatively:* Four-field technique by adding lateral portals for which borders are:
  - Anterior margin—Symphysis pubis
  - Posterior margin covers 50% of rectum in IB
  - Sacral hollow S_2-S_3 interspace in advanced disease.
  - Superior margin—Inferior edge of L_4
  - Inferior margin—Inferior edge of ischium.
  - Beam energy—use four-fields when using cobalt or 4–6 MV
  - X-rays—15–18 MV X-rays.

Dose Prescription

Sequencing of EBRT and ICRT

- In higher stage disease EBRT is used prior to ICRT to shrink the tumor and bring it close to radioactive sources
- In lower stage disease 40 Gy/4 weeks/20 # @ 200c Gy/# + 20–25 Gy to point A with LDR
- In higher stage disease 50 Gy/5 weeks/25#@200 cGy/# with introduction of a midline shield after 40 Gy
- Followed by ICRT 25–30 Gy to point A by single LDR application or 21–25 Gy to point A in 3–4# by HDR
- Concurrent chemotherapy to be considered with EBRT.

Patient Care

Skin reaction in sacral and perineal regions is common. Exposure to air and keeping skin dry. One percent hydrocortisone cream reduces erythema and irritation. Low residue diet. Diarrhea is treated when necessary. If severe interrupt treatment or reduce dose per fraction.

IRRADIATION OF REGIONAL LYMPHATICS ONLY

When ICRT has been Done Prior to EBRT

- Portal same as pelvic field with central shielding with rectangular blocks or step wedge (following lateral fall off dose of ICRT).

Width of shield: – 3–4 cm

– 3 cm when dose up to 20 Gy given

– 4 cm when 20–25 Gy remaining.

If block inserted before 40 Gy, then should not extend to the top of the field (may shield common iliac and presacral nodes).

Persistent Parametrial Tumor (Residual Parametrial Disease)

- Additional 10 Gy in 5–6# by reduced AP/PA portals:
  - If unilateral—8 × 12 cm (field as pelvic field)

– If bilateral—12 × 12 cm portal (with midline shielding to protect bladder and rectum).

Para-aortic Nodal Irradiation

Position—Supine.

Borders

Superior: T12-L1 interspace.
Inferior: Above pelvic field with adequate gap between two fields.
Width: 9–10 cm (determined with CT/IVP, etc.).

Spinal cord dose (from T12-L2) should be kept below 45 Gy by interposing 2 cm wide HVL shield in posterior portal after delivery of 32–46 Gy.

CARCINOMA VAGINA

Role of Radiation Therapy

It is the treatment of choice.

Assessment of Primary Tumor

Clinical assessment (bimanual P/V, P/R)
- Multiple biopsies
- Dilatation and curettage
- Cervical biopsies
- FNAC palpable LN
- CT scan.

Target Delineation

Target defined by:
- Barium swab in vagina
- Barium in rectum
- Introitus marker.

Target Volume
- Vagina and pelvic lymph nodes
- Inguinal lymph nodes in distal vaginal involvement.

Radiotherapy Technique

Field Placements

Borders
- *Superior:* L_5-S_1 junction
- *Inferior:* Beyond distal end of tumor defined by the marker or bead
- *Lateral:* 2 cm beyond pelvic brim
- If inguinal lymph nodes are to be boosted—direct appositional field used.

Alternatively, Four-field technique

Beam energy—Telecobalt

10–18 MV photons (with unequal loading)

Or 6 MV X-ray anteriorly and 18 MV photons posteriorly to achieve higher inguinal lymph node dose.

Dose Prescription

- 40 Gy/20#/4 weeks@ 2Gy/#

  Followed by boost 25 Gy at 0.5 cm from either by the surface of the applicator in ICRT or at 85% reference isodose curve in interstitial RT
- Or 20–24 Gy/10–12# in 2–2.5 week with EBRT.

Patient Care

Skin reaction in sacral and perineal regions is common. Exposure to air and keeping skin dry. 1% hydrocortisone cream reduces erythema and irritation. Low residue diet. Diarrhea is treated when necessary. If severe, interrupt treatment or reduce dose per fraction.

CARCINOMA VULVA

Role of Radiation Therapy

- Adjuvant vulvar irradiation to prevent local recurrence after surgery.
- Definitive vulvar irradiation with or without concurrent chemotherapy.
- Adjuvant nodal irradiation after nodal dissection.
- Definitive nodal irradiation with or without concurrent chemotherapy.

Assessment of Primary Tumor

Clinical assessment and local examination. CT/MRI to assess depth of inguinal nodes.

Target Delineation

Target Volume

- Vulva
- Bilateral groins
- Lower pelvic nodes.

Radiotherapy Technique

Medium/high energy photons in AP/PA oppositional portal Position-supine with thighs straight or in frog-leg position (minimizes bolus effect of skin folds).

Field Placements

Borders

- *Superior:* Middle of sacroiliac joint/L5-S1 interspace:
  - If pelvic lymph nodes positive, L3-L4 interspace.

- *Inferior:* Entire vulva and most superficial inguinal lymph nodes (about 6–8 cm inferior to inguinal skin crease).
- *Lateral:* 2 cm lateral to widest part in pelvic inlet (should extend out to anterior superior iliac spine to include inguinal ligament) Alternatively—Four-field technique
  Beam energy—18 MV photons with anterior loading.
- 18 MeV electrons to boost inguinal lymph nodes.

Dose Prescription

- Nodal irradiation 45–50 Gy/5 weeks/25fx
- If ulcerated and fixed-64–68 Gy
- Adjuvant vulvar irradiation 45–50 Gy/5 weeks/22–25 fx
- Definitive vulvar irradiation
- Small tumors < 4 cm—58–62 Gy with concurrent chemotherapy
- Larger inoperable tumors—64–72 Gy, if surgery not contemplated.

Patient Care

Skin reaction in sacral and perineal regions is common. Exposure to air and keeping skin dry. One percent hydrocortisone cream reduces erythema and irritation. Low residue diet. Diarrhea is treated when necessary. If severe, interrupt treatment or reduce dose per fraction.

CARCINOMA OVARY

Role of Radiation Therapy

Adjuvant treatment may be warranted due to risk of transcoelomic spread. But role of RT is debatable in view of increased abdominal toxicity and better outcome of modern adjuvant chemotherapy.

- Presently whole abdominal irradiation is being investigated with use of tomotherapy/volumetric arc IMRT to minimize toxicity.

- Historical methods like moving strip/Martinez technique are being explained for benefit of students.

Target Delineation

Target volume: Entire peritoneal cavity from diaphragm to pelvic floor.

Radiotherapy Technique

Field placements: Parallel opposing fields.
Various techniques: • Strip technique (MDAH 1950s)
                        • Martinez technique
                        • Modified Martinez technique.

Appositional AP/PA Portals Borders

- *Superior:* 1.5–2 cm (above diaphragm)
- *Inferior:* Inferior border of obturator foramen
- *Lateral:* Whole peritoneum with a margin of subcutaneous tissue
- Kidney to be protected after 15 Gy by shielding.

Localization

Simulator films taken with patient in supine position at an extended FSD to obtain required field size. If at an extended SSD the posterior field cannot be treated, then the patient is treated prone. IVP helps to assess location and function of kidney. It also helps in making shields. Shielding also added inferiorly to protect femurs and subcutaneous tissues.

Pelvis boosted with pelvic fields as in carcinoma cervix (described elsewhere).

Dose Prescription

25–30 Gy in 20 fx/4 weeks + pelvic boost-20 Gy/10#/2 weeks.

Martinez Technique

Open Fields with Special Design

1. Treatment delivered with series of AP/PA opposed fields beginning with RT to pelvis.

Borders

- *Superior:* L5 vertebral level
- *Inferior:* Lower border of obturator foramen.

2. Then extended to entire abdomen and pelvic peritoneum extending to 1.5 cm above diaphragm for 20#/1.5 Gy for 4 weeks.
   - After 20 Gy kidneys are shielded (either by full thickness block in posterior field or 50% transmission block in both fields).
   - After 15 Gy 50% transmission block placed in both fields to shield liver.

3. Last field is continuous pelvic and para-aortic and partial diaphragmatic T-shaped field for 8# of 1.5 Gy in 10 days.

Dosage

Whole peritoneum receives 30 Gy/20#

Pelvis	51 Gy/33#
Liver	22.5 Gy/23#
Kidneys	20 Gy/20#

MODIFIED MARTINEZ TECHNIQUE

Used in patients with suspected bowel compromise:

Whole abdomen receives	22 Gy/17#
Diaphragmatic boost	15 Gy
Pelvic boost	24 Gy by four-field technique as in carcinoma cervix
	Para-aortic boost omitted

Patient Care

Recommend ondansetron 8 mg one hour before and 3 hours after radiotherapy. Skin reaction in sacral and perineal region are common. Exposure to air and keeping skin dry. One percent hydrocortisone cream reduces erythema and irritation. Low residue diet. Diarrhea is treated when necessary. If severe, interrupt treatment or reduce dose per fraction.

OVARIAN ABLATION

Decline in ovarian function is slower by radiotherapy than that by surgical ablation/removal.
Fields: AP/PA portals after locating ovary by CT scan/USG (**Fig. 3.2**).
Superior margin: L5.
Inferior margin: Middle of femoral heads.
Lateral margins: 1 cm lateral to pelvic wall.

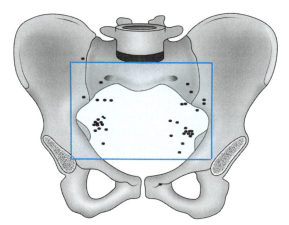

Fig. 3.2 Target volume for radiation menopause showing variable position of the ovaries

Portal size: 12 × 12 cm.

Dosage: 15 Gy/5#/over 5 days.

Dosage required for ablation is age dependent and higher in younger patients.

MALIGNANCY DURING PREGNANCY

Treatment depends on many factors:

1. Period of gestation
2. Type, location, size, and stage of the cancer
3. The wishes of the expectant mother and family.

As some treatments can harm the fetus, especially in the first trimester, treatment may be delayed until the second or third trimesters. When cancer is diagnosed later in pregnancy, one should wait to start treatment until the baby is born, or even consider inducing labor early. In some cases, such as early stage cervical cancer we wait to treat the cancer until after delivery.

Staging imaging tests should be limited to those associated with the lowest exposure to ionizing radiation. Abdominal radiography isotope scans, and computerized tomography should be avoided. Magnetic resonance imaging, ultrasound, and biopsies are considered safe during pregnancy. When possible, a lead shield covering the abdomen offers extra protection to the fetus. The use of radiopharmaceutical agents for bone, liver, and pulmonary scans require the interruption of breastfeeding for a period depending on isotope and its dosage. The radionuclide that has the shortest excretion time in breast milk should be used.

The management of each pregnant patient diagnosed with a malignancy has to be individualized and involves a multidisciplinary team of medical personnel. The patient and her family need counseling regarding the diagnosis, long-term prognosis, options of termination of pregnancy, choice of chemotherapeutic agents and their effects on the fetus and pregnancy. There is no entirely safe cytotoxic drug or timing of exposure for the developing fetus.

The administration of chemotherapy during pregnancy will not always produce a poor outcome. With the proper attention and a high index of suspicion, most of tumors can be detected early. Even with those negative prognostic attributes and characteristics, tumors still can be treated successfully and the patients can go on to lead productive lives.

CHAPTER 4

Carcinoma of Breast

Kanika Sharma

ROLE OF RADIATION THERAPY

Indications of Chest Wall Radiation

- Positive resection margin or gross residual disease
- T3 tumors and T4 tumor
- Four or more positive nodes in axilla
- Close surgical margins
- Lymphovascular invasion
- 1–3 lymph node in presence of other risk factors.

Indications of Axillary Irradiation

- Four or more axillary lymph node positive
- Perinodal disease
- Inadequate surgical dissection (less than 10 lymph nodes dissected)
- Unknown axillary status
- Posterior axillary boost needed in obese patients where anterior field is unable to deliver adequate dose to axillary nodes as in patients with separation >12 cm and where axilla is heavily involved.

Assessment of Primary Tumor

Clinical examination and diagrammatic documentation of primary tumor and nodal areas.

- Mammography
- MRI breast
- Grossing of surgical specimen for size, site and extent
- Histology for size, type, grade, margin receptor status and lymph node status
- Extent of surgical scar.

TARGET DELINEATION

Target Volume

- *In intact breast:* Entire breast with chest wall with one cm margin and a small portion of underlying lung
- *In operated cases:* Radiopaque surgical clips placed per-operatively at margins of tumor bed assist in defining target volume. After modified radical mastectomy—chest wall and small portion of underlying lung.

Radiotherapy Technique

Planning is individualized to accommodate topographic features:

- Whole breast technique (as after BCT and for LABC after neoadjuvant chemotherapy showing good regression of disease)
- Locoregional RT technique chest wall, axilla and SCF.

Patient Positioning

Supine with arm abducted at 90°. Immobilization devices such as alpha cradle and plastic molds may be used. Slope of the chest wall can be corrected with triangular wedge or incline under head and shoulders.

Field Placements

Whole Breast Technique

Medial and lateral tangential portals:

- *Upper border:* Lower margin of clavicle or intercostal space
- *Medial border:* At or over 1 cm over midline

- *Lateral border:* 2 cm beyond all palpable breast tissue (Midaxillary line)
- *Inferior border:* 2 cm below inframammary fold.

Locoregional RT

- *Upper border:* 2nd intercostal space (angle of Louis)
- *Medial border:* At or 1 cm over midline. Abuts lateral margin of IMN field if used
- *Lateral border:* Midaxillary line
- *Inferior border:* 2 cm below inframammary fold.

Axilla, Supraclavicular and Infraclavicular Field

Direct Field

- *Upper border:* In the neck to cover supraclavicular fossa across curve of shoulder till thyrocricoid groove.
- *Medial border:* 1 cm to contralateral side at level of sternal notch extending upwards following medial border of sterno-cleidomastoid muscle to thyrocricoid groove.
- *Lateral border:* If axilla not heavily infiltrated, at acromioclavicular joint. If axilla heavily infiltrated, at deltopectoral groove.
- *Inferior border:* Abuts upper border of tangential fields.
  The head of humerus and acromioclavicular joint is shielded.

Internal Mammary Nodal Portal

Not being routinely used. Consideration should be given for tumors of central and medial quadrant, and locally advanced breast cancers.

Direct Fields

Borders
- *Upper border:* Inferior border of SC field.
- Medial border midline (2 cm across midline).

- *Lateral border:* 6 cm from and parallel to medial border (4 cm to ipsilateral side).
- *Inferior border:* Base of xiphoid.

Posterior Axillary Boost Portal

Patient Positioning

Prone with head turned to contralateral side, forearm rotated down shoulder in contact with table top back of hand on pelvic brim.

Borders

- *Medial superior:* Follows spine of scapula.
- *Lateral superior:* Bisects head of humerus.
- *Lower lateral:* Medial to border of latissimus dorsi.
- *Inferior:* Match inferior border of anterior field 1.5–2 cm lung tissue is included medially along concavity of bony thorax.
- *Beam energy:*   Cobalt
                   6 MV X-rays
                   8–15 MeV electrons

Dose Prescription

- *Primary:* 50 Gy/25 fractions/5 weeks at a dose rate of 2 Gy/ day treated 5 days a week. Dose calculated at mid separation 3–3.5 cm within the flap.
- *Regional nodes:* 50 Gy/25 fractions/5 weeks at dose rate of 2 Gy/day treated 5 days a week

  Dose calculated at 3 cm depth for IMN field and 0.5 cm for SCF field.

  At midplane 2 cm below midportion of clavicle in posterior axillary field.

  In patients with breast conservation, boost is given to lumpectomy cavity either by:

- Elecrons or photons 15–18 Gy in 6–7 fractions
- Interstitial brachytherapy 20–25 Gy at 85% isodose in 3–4 days.

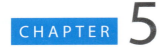

Gastrointestinal Tract Tumors

Kanika Sharma

ESOPHAGUS

Role of Radiation Therapy

- Definitive as radiation therapy alone especially in cervical esophagus.
- *Postoperative:* When resected margin positive
  Tumor infiltration into mucosa
  Positive mediastinal LN.
- Preoperative in T3, T4 and node positive tumors.

Assessment of Primary Tumor

- Barium swallow
- Upper GI endoscopy
- Contrast-enhanced computer tomography (CECT) thorax and abdomen, endoscopic ultrasound.

Target Delineation

Target volume 5 cm proximal and 5 cm distal margin beyond primary tumor, 2.5 cm radial margin and regional nodes.

Patient Position

Supine with arms up.

Radiotherapy Technique

Portals: AP/PA until cord tolerance and then treated with either lateral or oblique fields which avoid the spinal cord.

Another option is to treat the patient with a three-field technique (AP and posterior obliques), with at least one field not contributing to spinal cord dose.

Borders

- *Superior:* 5 cm above uppermost extent of disease. Can be decreased to 3 cm in case of 3 DCRT/IMRT.
- *Inferior:* 5 cm below lowermost extent of disease.
- *Lateral:* 2.5 cm either side beyond tumor (radial margin) or 1 cm radial margin in case of CT based planning (for PTV).

Three Field Technique

AP/PA—same as described earlier.

Then **three fields**.

Anterior field same.

Oblique field angles are determined by TPS or manually after contouring.

Three-dimensional treatment planning allows for further optimization of field shaping and orientation compared with two-dimensional (2D) techniques with use of wedge.

Intensity-modulated radiation therapy (IMRT) may be advantageous due to complex geometric target of these cancers and the potential benefits of more conformal treatment with regard to normal organ toxicity. However, there are limitations due to respiratory and cardiac motion.

Intraluminal Brachytherapy

For delivery of localized boost after EBRT or as palliative treatment.

- Dose in palliative 15 Gy at 1 cm from center of axis of source.
- Dose in boost—7.5 Gy at start and end of treatment.
- Dose is prescribed at 1 cm from center of axis of source.

Dose Prescription

1. Definitive

Radical 39.6 Gy/22#/4.2 weeks @1.8 Gy/# with concurrent chemotherapy.

Boost till 50.4 Gy 30/#/6 weeks in 6.3 weeks @1.8 Gy/# after spine sparing with 3 fields.

2. Palliative

20 Gy/5#/5 days by opposed AP-PA portals.

3. Preoperative

45 Gy/25 fraction (#)/5 weeks @1.8 Gy per # with concurrent chemotherapy after which surgery is planned.

Patient Care

Esophagitis is inevitable, treated with dispersible aspirin and mucaine gel. Antifungals are also warranted.

STOMACH

Role of Radiation Therapy

- Technically unresectable
- Medically unfit
- Incomplete tumor resection/gross residual disease
- Positive margins
- Transmural invasion
- Regional lymph node positivity
- Preoperative.

Assessment of Primary Tumor

- Endoscopic ultrasonography
- CT abdomen with oral and intravenous contrast

- PET scan
- Simulation (supine with arms up).

Target Delineation

Target Volume

- Gastric/tumor bed (with preoperative CT/postoperative CT scan with surgical clips).
- Anastomosis and gastric remnant.
- *Regional lymphatics*: Along lesser and greater curvature, celiac axis, pancreaticoduodenal, suprapancreatic, porta hepatic, splenic nodes (in proximal stomach involvement).
- Para-aortic till level of mid L_3.

Radiotherapy Technique

Field Placements (Fig. 5.1)

- *Upper border*: Bottom of T_8/T_9 to cover celiac axis, GE junction, fundus and dome of diaphragm.
- *Lower border*: Bottom of L_3 to cover gastroduodenal nodes.
- *Left border*: Includes 2/3rd to 3/4th of left hemidiaphragm to cover fundus, supradiaphragmatic nodes and splenic nodes.
- *Right border*: 3–4 cm lateral to vertebral bodies to cover antrum, porta hepatic and gastroduodenal nodes.

Dose Prescription

45 Gy/5 weeks@1.8 Gy/#.

Field reduction at 45 Gy to deliver 50.4 Gy with reduced field with multiple fields.

Intraoperative—10–35 Gy to tumor bed excluding or protecting surrounding structures.

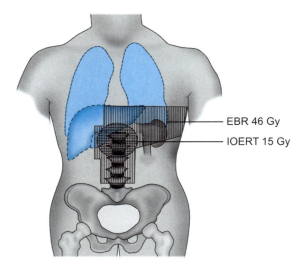

Fig. 5.1 Combination of external beam radiation (EBR) and intraoperative electron irradiation (IOERT) in a gastric cancer patient

Patient Care

Recommend ondansetron 8 mg one hour before and 3 hours after radiotherapy. Avoid oily and spicy food. Avoid heavy meal. 1–2 hours before radiation therapy, calcium and B complex supplementation is required for 2–3 months after RT.

RECTUM

Role of Radiation Therapy

- Preoperative in locally advanced tumors which are considered unresectable.
- Adjuvant in patients with T4 tumors and selected T3 tumors and positive lymph nodes.

Assessment of Primary Tumor

- Digital examination
- Sigmoidoscopy
- Colonoscopy
- Double contrast barium enema
- Endorectal USG
- CT scan
- MRI.

Target Delineation

Target Volume

- Primary tumor
- Tumor bed
- Adjacent lymph nodes
- Presacral region.

The CTV encompasses all the perirectal tissue, presacral space and lymphatics of the internal iliac chain.

In the postoperative setting, the entire preoperative tumor bed must be reconstructed and included within the CTV (often identified separately as a boost volume). Preoperative imaging, operative reports and surgical clip placement should be reviewed.

Radiotherapy Technique

Simulation

The anal verge should be marked with a radiopaque marker and rectal contrast instilled into the rectum to assist radiographic identification of the primary lesion. Patients who have undergone abdominoperineal resection must have the perineal scar marked and included in the initial pelvic fields, with appropriate bolus utilized posteriorly.

Position: Prone, ensure bladder full, use of belly board.

Field Placements

AP/PA, 2 lateral and 2 posterior obliques, 4 field plan.

Borders

Whole Pelvis PA

- *Superior*: L5/S1.
- *Inferior*: 3 cm below initial tumor volume or inferior obturator foramen (extending from top sacrum to 5 cm below primary tumor bed).

   If there is high-risk of tumor recurrence in the perineum then lower border should cover perineal scar. The perineal scar must be included in the initial fields for patients who have undergone abdominoperineal resection.
- *Lateral*: 1.5 cm outside lateral pelvis (to include pelvic side walls and internal iliac nodes).
- *Posteriorly*: Presacral lymph node and sacral hollow are covered anteriorly with adequate margin.

Lateral

- *Posterior*: Behind the sacrum.
- *Anterior*:
  - Posterior pubic symphysis for T3 lesions.
  - Anterior pubic symphysis pubis for T4 lesions.
  - Boost-tumor + 2–3 cm margins.

   The GTV should be boosted with reduced fields including the tumor with a 2–3 cm margin. Separate boost fields for involved inguinal lymph nodes are needed. Boosting the primary lesion with a perineal field precludes CT planning in the treatment position and should be reserved for tumors that can be completely exposed to ensure coverage (e.g. tumors of the anal margin).

   When performing conformal radiotherapy the CTV should extend superiorly to include the sacral promontory, posteriorly to include the anterior wall of the sacrum, and laterally include vasculature and presacral soft tissue to the border of the iliopsoas muscles and entire mesorectal fascia.

In the mid pelvis, include perirectal fat anterior to the rectum. In addition, 1–2 cm of posterior bladder or uterus may be included if at risk of subclinical extension of disease for patients who have adjacent, locally advanced lesions.

In the lower pelvis, the CTV includes all the perirectal fat inferiorly and laterally extending to the levator ani muscles. It should include the posterior wall of the prostate or vagina as well. A larger margin of anterior pelvic organs is indicated for tumors with documented invasion (T4). The CTV should also include 2 cm of normal rectum above and below the primary tumor.

Dose Prescription

Preoperative

44 Gy/22#/4.5 weeks followed by surgery at 6–8 weeks in fixed tumors or 25 Gy/5#/1 week followed immediately by surgery in mobile tumors.

Postoperative

45–50 Gy/25#/5 weeks @1.8 Gy/#

If residual macroscopic disease-boost 10–15 Gy/5–7#/1.2 weeks to a total dose of 55–60 Gy in 6.5–7 weeks.

Inoperable or Recurrent Disease

45–50 Gy/20–25#/4–5 weeks.

Patient Care

Skin reaction in sacral and perineal region is common. Exposure to air and keeping skin dry. One percent hydrocortisone cream reduces erythema and irritation. Low residue diet. Diarrhea is treated when necessary. If severe, interrupt treatment or reduce dose per fraction. Advice usage of surgical air cushion for sitting to decrease perineal reactions.

COLON

Role of Radiation Therapy

Preoperative in unresectable tumors.

Adjuvant in selected T3, T4 tumors, and positive lymph nodes. Radiotherapy may not be required in view of combination chemotherapy in most cases.

Assessment of Primary Tumor

- Sigmoidoscopy
- Colonoscopy
- Double contrast barium enema
- CT scan
- MRI.

Target Delineation

Target Volume

The tumor bed and adjacent pelvic and retroperitoneal lymphatics.

Radiotherapy Technique

Patients treated with radiotherapy for colon cancer are treated with the principles as rectal cancer. The initial CTV generally includes the tumor bed and adjacent pelvic/retroperitoneal lymphatics, with a subsequent boost to the tumor bed (or tumor preoperatively). Preoperative imaging, operative reports and identification of surgical clips demarcating the tumor bed are essential to define targets and design fields.

Dose Prescription

Preoperative

- 44 Gy/22#—surgery after 6–8 weeks
- 20 Gy/5#/1 week—1 week later surgery for mobile tumors.

Postoperative

- 40–50/25#/5 weeks
- If residual macroscopic disease—10–15 Gy/5–7# for small volume to total dose 55–60 Gy in 6.5–7 weeks.

Patient Care

Low residue diet. Antiemetics and antidiarrheals.

ANAL CANAL

Role of Radiation Therapy

Definitive Treatment

Abdominoperineal resection is reserved as salvage treatment for patients with persistent or recurrent disease after radiotherapy.

Assessment of Primary Tumor

- Inspection of perineal skin.
- Digital rectal examination for extent of tumor.
- Vaginal examination to detect involvement of posterior vaginal wall.
- Transrectal ultrasound for depth of tumor.
- Proctoscopy and sigmoidoscopy to define upper limit of tumor and biopsy.
- Double contrast–barium enema to exclude synchronous lesion in colon.

Target Delineation

Target volume includes the primary tumor, clinically involved lymph nodes, as well as perianal tissues and regional lymphatics at risk for subclinical spread of the disease.

The clinical target volumes (CTVs) include inguinal-pelvic lymphatics and perianal tissues. Adjacent to the primary anal tumor, the CTV should include a 1–2 cm radial margin of surrounding soft tissue. Longitudinally, it should include any portions of the anal canal not involved in the tumor. The CTV also includes the inguinal and pelvic lymph nodes.

Radiotherapy Technique

Simulation

To reduce skin toxicity, cutaneous folds within the medial groin may be minimized by moderately abducting the patient's legs and using an immobilization device to ensure set-up reproducibility of the lower extremities. The clinical extent of any visible or palpable perianal tumor should be demarcated with radiopaque markers as it may not be apparent on simulation imaging. The anal verge should also be marked and the rectum may be visualized with rectal contrast.

Treatment position: Supine, with urinary bladder full.

Field Placements

Borders
- Initial large fields AP/PA
  - *Superior:* L5/S1
  - *Inferior:* 2.5 cm on anus
  - *Lateral:* 2 cm lateral to greater sciatic notch
- Reduced field
  - AP/PA

– Superior border-Inferior border of sacroiliac joints till 40 Gy
– Reduced to boost original tumor + 2–2.5 cm till 55–59 Gy for T3-T4.

Dose Prescription

Initial Target Volume

40–45 Gy/20–25#//4–5 weeks @1.8 Gy/#.

Boost either by

1. Interstitial implantation—20–25 Gy to 85% reference isodose curve.
2. EBRT—20–25 Gy/10–13#/2–2.5 weeks to give total dose of 60–65 Gy in 6.5–7 weeks to primary tumor.

Patient Care

Skin reaction in sacral and perineal region are common. Exposure to air and keeping skin dry. One percent hydrocortisone cream reduces erythema and irritation. Low residue diet. Diarrhea is treated when necessary. If severe, interrupt treatment or reduce dose per fraction. Advice usage of surgical air cushion for sitting to decrease perineal reactions.

PANCREAS

Role of Radiation Therapy

- Is debatable
- *Several options:*
  – Postoperative setting where node positive and positive resection margins.

- Patients with unresectable cancers who have a favorable functional status should be considered for chemoradiotherapy.
- Preoperative chemoradiotherapy, is not established as a treatment standard by prospective randomized trial but has been increasingly being used in borderline operable tumors.

Assessment of Primary Tumor

- CT scan (contrast enhanced)
- MRI scan.

Target Delineation

- Ideally titanium clips assist in defining treatment volume
- Portal film/simulator—supine with renal contrast and contrast in stomach and duodenal loop.

Target Volume

Preoperative tumor volume with lymph nodes (1–2 cm margin).

- *Head*: Pancreaticoduodenal, suprapancreatic and celiac nodes, porta hepatic, enteroduodenal loop and tumor with 2 cm margin.
- *Body/tail*: Treat pancreaticoduodenal, porta hepatic, lateral suprapancreatic, nodes of splenic hilum and gross tumor with 2–3 cm margin.

Simulation

Patients are generally simulated in the supine position with arms extended over the head using a wingboard or similar device to ensure reproducibility and to allow treatment of oblique or lateral fields. If treatment fields will encompass any stomach, the patient should be both simulated and treated with an empty stomach (minimum 4 hours) to reduce gastric distension and improve target reproducibility.

Radiotherapy Technique

Position: Supine with arms up with oral contrast and renal contrast to delineate kidneys.

Field Placements

Four-field technique with disproportionate weighting of the anterior and posterior fields to reduce dose to the liver from the lateral fields.

AP/PA:
- *Superior:* T10/T11.
- *Inferior:* L3/L4.
- *Left border:* 2 cm to the left of the edge of vertebral body or 2 cm from the tumor (or past the splenic hilum for pancreatic tail lesions).
- *Right border:* Preoperative location of duodenum (to cover the duodenum and portahepatic).

    With the lateral fields, these boundaries should be customized on the basis of patient differences in target volumes as well as normal structure location.

Lateral: Anterior margin 1.5–2 cm beyond gross disease.

    Posterior margin block the cord but cover 1.5–2 cm of the vertebral body (the posterior border generally splits the vertebral bodies, while the anterior border is placed at least 2 cm anterior to the tumor, maintaining a 3–4 cm margin anterior to the vertebral bodies to ensure coverage of para-aortic lymph nodes).

    Cone down to gross tumor + 2 cm margin at 45 Gy (Boost fields encompass unresected tumor or original tumor bed with 1.5–2 cm margins).

    IMRT for pancreatic cancers provides dosimetric advantages and controls dose to bowel.

Dose Prescription

45 Gy/25 #/5 weeks @1.8 Gy/#

    With additional boost to complete 56 Gy/28#/5½ weeks treated 5 days a week. The final dose depends on treatment volume patients general condition and whether concomitant chemotherapy is administered.

Palliative Treatment

40–50 Gy/20–25#/4–5 weeks@ 2 Gy/#.

Patient Care

Nausea, vomiting and diarrhea are common. Oral medication and adequate hydration are required. Treatment is suspended, if side effects are severe.

HEPATOBILIARY

HEPATOCELLULAR CARCINOMA

Role of Radiotherapy

- Unresectable tumors
- As palliative in multiple lesions
- Medically inoperable.

Assessment of Primary Tumor

- CT scan
- MRI scan.

Target Delineation

Target Volume

Preoperative tumor volume with a margin.

Radiotherapy Technique

Position: Supine with arms over head, use wingboard and alpha cradle.

Field Placements

AP/PA portals based on CT scan.
- CTV—Gross tumor with 1 cm margin in all directions.
- PTV—CTV + 0.5 cm for set-up error +3 cm for organ motion.

Dose Prescription

Conventional at least 55 Gy
SBRT — Radical – 4 Gy/fraction to a total dose of 52 Gy
      — Palliative – 21–30 Gy in 3 Gy per fraction.

Patient Care

Oral medication and adequate hydration are required. Treatment is suspended, if side effects are severe.

GALLBLADDER

Role of Radiation Therapy

- Positive margins
- LN involvement
- Neural invasion
- Residual tumor
- Inadequate surgery.

Assessment of Primary Tumor

Target Delineation

Target volume: Preoperative tumor volume and lymph nodes with 1–2 cm margin.

Radiotherapy Technique

Position: Supine with arms over head.

Use wingboard to immobilize arms to stabilize arms and alpha cradle to stabilize torso.

Field Placements

CT scan based preoperative tumor volume and lymph nodes with 1–2 cm margin. Additional margin of 0.5 cm for set-up error and 3 cm margin for organ motion.

Boost by EBRT or IORT.

Dose Prescription

- 45 Gy/25#/5 weeks@1.8 Gy/#
- Boost to tumor bed to 60 Gy total.

Patient Care

Oral medication and adequate hydration are required. Treatment is suspended, if side effects are severe.

CHOLANGIOCARCINOMA

Role of Radiotherapy

- Nonresectable tumors
- Incompletely resected tumors.

Target Delineation

- USG right upper abdomen
- MRI scan
- ERCP.

Treatment volume: Volume-tumor with lymph nodes (1–2 cm margin).

Radiotherapy Technique

Position: Supine with arms over chest.

Portal: AP/PA or multiple fields CT scan based.

Cover tumor bed, porta hepatic and celiac axis + 1.5 cm margin. Consider extending field 3–5 cm into liver to cover additional intrahepatic bile duct length, additional margin for organ motion (3 cm).

Dose Prescription

In resectable tumor, 45 Gy/25 #/5 weeks with additional boost by EBRT to deliver 60 Gy after cone down, ^{192}Ir brachytherapy (20–25Gy).
IORT at time of surgery.
In unresectable tumor, 20 Gy/5 #/week.

Patient Care

Oral medication and adequate hydration are required. Treatment is suspended, if side effects are severe.

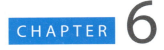

Thoracic Tumors

Vikash Kumar

LUNG CANCER

Small Cell Lung Cancer

Role of Radiotherapy

- *Limited disease:*
  - For T1N0 disease resection followed by chemotherapy is treatment of choice.
  - Combination chemotherapy (CDDP + Etoposide q3 weeks × 4 cycles) significantly increases survival and quality of life.
  - Consolidation radiotherapy concurrent with chemotherapy increases local control and survival in patients who achieve complete response after chemotherapy.
  - Prophylactic cranial irradiation reduces the risk of brain metastasis by 50%.
- *Extensive disease:*
  - Combination chemotherapy but complete remissions are usually shortlived.
  - Radiotherapy improves local control but does not improve survival and is recommended for palliation.

Definition of Target Volume

GTV + 1.5 cm margin which includes ipsilateral hilum, and bilateral mediastinum from thoracic inlet to subcarinal region

(5 cm below subcarinal region or adequate margin for subcarinal disease).

Dose Prescription

SCLC

Adjuvant RT (after chemotherapy): 45 Gy in 30 fractions given in 3 weeks (1.5 Gy/#; 2#/day) or up to 66–70 Gy in 2 Gy fractions if given once daily.

Porphylactic cranial irradiation: 25 Gy in 10 fractions given in 2 weeks, if complete or partial response to treatment.

Nonsmall Cell Lung Cancer

Role of Radiotherapy

- Patient with N+ disease, postoperative residual disease— radiotherapy improves locoregional control but does not improve survival.
- Patient unfit for surgery.
- Inoperable stage IIIA disease with good performance status may be treated with radical radiotherapy after induction chemotherapy.

  Stage IIIB disease (T3/N2-N3 bulky unresectable) intent of treatment is usually palliative.

Palliative Radiotherapy

- For symptomatic relief of dyspnea, dysphagia, hemoptysis or pain; irrespective of histological type.
- Brain/Bone metastasis.
- Inoperable pancoast tumor—requires high dose palliative radiotherapy.

General Guidelines

Stage I-II (Operable):
- Lobectomy is preferred over pneumonectomy, wedge resection in physiologically compromised patients.
- Adjuvant chemotherapy for completely resected tumor.
- For margin positive, nodal extracapsular extension postoperative RT followed by chemotherapy.

Stage I-II (Marginally operable):
- Preoperative chemotherapy → surgery → chemotherapy.
- For margin positive, nodal extracapsular extension postoperative radiotherapy.

Stage I-II (Inoperable):
- Definitive radiotherapy to primary +/– involved nodes.
- Chemotherapy can be used either as induction, concurrent and/or consolidation.

Stage III (Operable or Marginally operable):

NACT ⟶ Restaging ⟶ If stable disease; surgery ⟶ Chemotherapy. Postoperative radiotherapy for positive margins, nodal extracapsular extension

Or

Concurrent chemoradiotherapy 45 Gy ⟶ Restage ⟶ Surgery ⟶ +/– Chemotherapy

If disease remains unresectable after restaging; definitive concurrent chemoradiotherapy is advised.

Stage IIIA inoperable:

Concurrent CT + radiotherapy followed by adjuvant chemotherapy (preferably)

Or

Induction chemotherapy followed by concurrent CT + radiotherapy

Stage IIIB no pleural effusion:
Concurrent CT + radiotherapy followed by adjuvant chemotherapy
or,
Induction chemotherapy followed by concurrent CT + radiotherapy
If T4N0-1, surgery followed by chemotherapy +/– radiotherapy,
or chemotherapy +/– radiotherapy followed by surgery ⟶
Chemotherapy

Stage IIIB with pleural effusion: Local treatment – Pleurodesis, and
treated as stage IV disease.

Stage IV: Good performance status – chemotherapy +/– palliative
radiotherapy.
Poor performance status—Best supportive care.

Planning Technique

Assessment of Primary Disease

- Clinical examination
- Chest radiography
- CECT chest
- MRI for chest wall invasion and neurovascular bundle
  involvement in case of pancoast tumor
- Pulmonary function test
- PET scan especially for mediastinal diseases.

Definition of Target Volume

Radical Treatment

- *GTV* is gross primary and nodal disease including LN(s) ≥1 cm or
  with significant uptake on PET.
- *CTV:* GTV + 1–1.5 cm margin.
- *PTV:* 1 cm in transverse direction and 1.5–2 cm in vertical
  direction.

For boost field, only the primary tumor and ipsilateral hilar lymph node are included in the target volume, with margins added for movement. Supraclavicular fossa is treated in case of superior lobe primary or gross upper mediastinal disease. Contralateral hilar or supraclavicular treatment is avoided unless involved.

- Used in postoperative T1-2N0-1 incompletely resected tumors
- Patients with N2 disease
- Stage IIIA patients with good- prognosis
- Patients with operable disease not fit for surgery.

Palliative Treatment

The volume includes the primary tumor with margins of approximately 2 cm and adjacent lymph nodes.

Dose Prescription

Nonsmall Cell Lung Carcinoma

Adjuvant radiotherapy (after surgery): 50 Gy in 25 fractions given in 5 weeks.

Radical Radiotherapy

Primary tumor + mediastinum - 45–50 Gy @1.8–2.0 Gy/fraction. Boost to 60 Gy for close/+ve margins or to 66 Gy for gross disease.

Palliative Treatment

10 Gy single fraction.

Patient Care

Radiation esophagitis—Mucaine gel, Dispirin, Soft diet.
High calorie protein diet.

SUPERIOR SULCUS TUMOR

If operable; concurrent CT + radiotherapy (45 Gy) followed by surgery then chemotherapy.
If marginally operable; concurrent CT + radiotherapy (45 Gy) ⟶ reassessment, if operable ⟶ surgery then chemotherapy.
If unresectable; concurrent CT + radiotherapy (definitive).

Planning Technique

The treatment field includes the tumor, supraclavicular and adjacent mediastinal and hilar lymph node and the vertebral bodies to encompass tumor infiltration of neural exit foramina. Field arrangements and shielding should be such that spinal cord receives minimal dose.

Simulation

Patient lies in supine position with arms up. Immobilization is done with wingboard or alfa cradle. 3D-CRT/IMRT is preferred to improve therapeutic ratio. Field margins are defined and AP simulator films are taken. A correction factor of 0.2–0.3 is used to adjust for reduced attenuation in the lungs. Wedges and compensating filters may be needed.

For CT simulation; the patient lies supine with proper immobilization devices similar to the treatment position. Slice thickness 0.5 cm from larynx to L2 to include all lung volume. Critical organs of interest such as heart, lung esophagus and spinal cord are outlined. Beam's eye view is used to assist choice of direction, size and shape of beam.

Field Arrangements

Radical treatment: Primary field planning.

Parallel opposing AP/PA portal is frequently used. This arrangement gives some hotspots outside the treatment volume and some inhomogeneous distribution. Alternatively, a three-field or four-field arrangements is used.

Radical treatment: Boost field planning/single phase planning.

Three-field technique is usually used to minimize dose to the lungs and spinal cord. 3D-CRT/IMRT (**Figs 6.1 and 6.2**).

Implementation of Plan

Fields are treated isocentrically. Particular attention is given to spinal cord in treatment portal and proper beam modifying devices, beam angulations, beam weightage to keep dose within tolerance limits. Plan is verified on treatment simulator to see whether portals are adequately covering the tumor especially considering spinal cord.

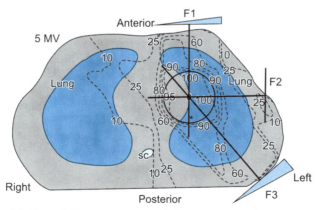

Fig. 6.1 Three-field arrangement with lung correction for treatment of lung lesion to give minimum dose to the spinal cord (sc). F1: Gantry 0°, 15° wedge, weight 120%, 8.5 × 9 cm; F2: Gantry 90°, weight 50%, 7.5 × 9 cm; F3: Gantry 140°, 45° wedge, weight 100%, 8.5 × 9 cm

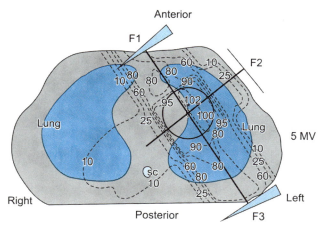

Fig. 6.2 Three-field arrangement with lung correction for treatment of lung lesion to give minimum dose to the contralateral lung. F1: Gantry 325°, 30° wedge, weight 100%, 8.5 × 9 cm; F2: Gantry 50°, weight 50%, 8 × 9 cm; F3: Gantry 145°, 30° wedge, weight 100%, 8.5 × 9 cm

Movement of Lung Tumors with Radiation

A movement of structures with respiration has a significant impact on the size, shape and position of PTV. Methods are:

   i. Gated radiotherapy
  ii. Active breathing control (ABC)
 iii. Image-guided radiotherapy (IGRT)
 iv. 4D-CT data acquisition and planning.

MESOTHELIOMA

Diagnostic Work-up

CXR, CT/MRI, PET for pleural thickening, effusions, mediastinal/chest wall/diaphragm involvement and pleural calcifications and histopathology for confirmation.

Treatment Recommendations

- *Stage I-II:* If resectable/N0, extrapleural pneumonectomy followed by RT after 3–6 weeks.
  If unresectable; chemotherapy.
- *Stage III-IV:* If resectable, treat as stage I-II, or with pemetrexed + cisplatin or with cisplatin and gemcitabine.

Radiation Techniques

Simulation

Patient in supine position with arms overhead.

Hemithoracic radiotherapy is planned 3–6 weeks after extrapleural pneumonectomy.

Conventional treatment: Parallel opposed AP/PA portals are used.

- *Upper margin:* Superior border of T1.
- *Lower margin:* Inferior border of L2.
- *Medial margin:* Contralateral edge of vertebral body, if mediastinum negative 1.5 cm beyond contralateral edge, if mediastinum is involved.
- *Lateral margin:* Flash along thoracic margins.

Part of liver and stomach is shielded throughout the treatment, humerus and heart are shielded after 20 Gy and spinal cord is shielded after 41.4 Gy. Scars are included within treatment field and are treated with bolus. Electron boost to the areas of chest wall shielded.

Dose Prescription

54 Gy in 30 fractions @ 1.8 Gy/#.

Electron beam therapy with appropriate energy is delivered concurrent with photon @ 1.5 Gy/#.

THYMOMA

Most common presentation is anterior mediastinal mass.

Diagnostic Work-up

- Histopathology
- CXR, CT chest
- β-hCG, AFP, LDH
- Anterior mediastinoscopy with biopsy.

Radiation Techniques

Simulation and Field Arrangements

Patient lies supine, usually; AP/PA portals are used 3D-CRT, if available should be used to decrease dose to the critical organs. Supraclavicular fossa is spared unless involved.
Lower border is extended 5 cm below carina to include mediastinum and a margin of 1–2 cm is added to obtain PTV.

Dose Prescription

- *Preoperative radiotherapy:* 1.8 Gy/# to 45 Gy
- *Stage II postoperative:* 1.8 Gy/# to 45 Gy
- *Stage III postoperative:* 1.8 Gy/# to 45–50 Gy
- *Gross residual disease:* 1.8 Gy/# to 54–60 Gy.

Dose Limitations

- Spinal cord <45 Gy
- Lung 70% <20 Gy
- Heart 70% <25–40 Gy
- Esophagus <60 Gy.

CHAPTER 7

Central Nervous System

Vikash Kumar

SUPPORTIVE CARE

Medical Decompression

Headache and/or vomiting (not severe): Dexamethasone 2 mg 8 hourly.

Headache and/or vomiting (not severe) with new or worsening neurological deficit—Dexamethasone 4 mg 8 hourly.

Headache and/or vomiting (severe) with deteriorating consciousness—Dexamethasone 8 mg 8 hourly with 20% Mannitol, 1 g/kg BW, 6–8 hourly.

Tapering of dexamethasone every 48 hrs.

Anticonvulsant Prophylaxis

Perioperative: For 4 weeks.

For patients who present with seizure: Continue for 2 years; discontinued if patients are seizure free for 2 years.

For patients who do not present with seizure: Usually not recommended. If access to medical care or close surveillance is lacking; prophylactic antiepileptic drug is continued for 2 years.

Phenytoin remains the most commonly used antiepileptic drug and being a microsomal enzyme inducer; should be used judiciously with chemotherapy. Levetiracetam, lamotrigine and pregabalin do not affect cytochrome P450 activity are now preferred.

GENERAL GUIDELINES FOR RADIATION THERAPY

- Following maximal safe resection; adjuvant radiotherapy is indicated for all high grade primary brain tumors.
- For completely excised benign tumors like pituitary adenomas, benign meningiomas and low-grade gliomas currently, there is no role of upfront adjuvant radiotherapy. Only surveillance is recommended.
- Radical radiotherapy is needed for tumors in eloquent cortex where only partial excision or biopsy is possible.
- Radiotherapy to start preferably 3–4 weeks after surgery.
- All patients to be planned by SAD technique only.
- Simulator based planning or marker films to be done.
- *Position:* Supine with appropriate neck flexion (neutral for frontoparietal and maximal flexion for temporal, sellar/ parasellar regions.
- Gross tumor volume (GTV) comprises contrast enhancing tumor on *preoperative* CT/MRI for all high-grade gliomas and any residual visible tumor on *postoperative* planning images for benign and low-grade tumors.
- *Immobilization of patients:* With orifit/uniframe casts.
- *Energy selection:*
    - Cobalt 60
    - 6 MV photons (15/18 MV when needed).
- All patients (except PCNSL) to be started on tablet dexamethasone 4 mg thrice daily and dose titrated subsequently (along with antacids).
- Antiseizure medications as indicated, therapeutic level is monitored.

Low-grade Glioma

Juvenile Pilocytic Astrocytoma

- *Gross total resection (GTR):* Observation.

- *Subtotal resection (STR):* Postoperative radiotherapy/SRS depending on tumor location, symptoms and age of patients.

Oligoastrocytoma, Oligodendroglioma, Astrocytomas Grade I and II

- *Gross total resection (GTR)/Subtotal resection (STR):* Observation if age <40 years.
  Immediate postoperative radiotherapy; delays time to relapse.
- *Target volumes:*
  GTV — T1 enhancement or FLAIR
  CTV — GTV + 1–2 cm margin.
- *EBRT:* 59.4 Gy in 33 fractions (1.8 Gy per fraction).

High-grade Glioma

Includes anaplastic astrocytoma, glioblastoma multiforme (GBM), anaplastic oligodendroglioma and anaplastic ependymoma.

Gross total resection/Subtotal resection followed by:

EBRT: 60 Gy in 30 fractions concurrent with temozolomide 75 mg/m^2 followed by adjuvant TMZ 200 mg/m^2 × 6 cycles (for GBM only and anaplastic astrocytoma) (150 mg /m^2 for 1st cycle).

40 Gy in 15 fractions for age ≥60 and KPS >50.

30 Gy in 10 fractions for age ≥65 and KPS <50.

Target Volume

Primary Field	GTV - T1 Enhancement + T2 flair.
	CTV - GTV + 2 cm margin
	PTV - 0.5 cm
	Boost Volume - GTV-T1 Enhancement.
	CTV - GTV + 2 cm margin

The most important part of the management of patients with GBM is effective supportive care. This includes treatment of cerebral edema with a potent glucocorticosteroid (dexamethasone);

seizure prophylaxis and therapy with a modern anticonvulsant; and rehabilitative care as physical, occupational, speech therapy, and emotional and psychological support is very essential.

Brainstem Glioma

About 70–80% are high-grade determined by MRI features and presentation.

Surgery is most appropriate in tumors of cervicomedullary junction, dorsal exophytic tumors protruding into IV ventricle, cystic tumors, enhancing tumors with clear margins that exert a space occupying effect.

Pontine tumors are the most common variety of brainstem tumor. They carry the worst prognosis; median survival is 9–12 months even with treatment. Biopsy and/or surgery is not recommended for diagnosis or treatment of intrinsic pontine or tectal gliomas and is not required.

Focal radiotherapy is the mainstay of treatment of brainstem glioma. There is role of temozolomide.

Target Volumes

Tumor with 2 cm margin or entire brainstem (up to C2) and any cerebellar extension with margin.

EBRT

60 Gy in 30 fractions for focal lesion.
For diffuse lesion; PTV include whole brainstem.
Dose limited to 54 Gy/30 fractions.

Important Note for Brainstem
Glioma and for Brainstem in CNS Irradiation

- If non-modulated beams are used; Dmax to brainstem should be limited to less than 55 Gy

- If intensity modulated beams are used, then Dmax to entire brainstem should be limited to below 56 Gy and dose to less than 1% volume limited below 59 Gy.

Optic Nerve Glioma

- Five percent of all CNS tumors in the pediatric age group.
- *Subdivided into:* Optic nerve gliomas, chiasmatic gliomas, and chiasmatic/hypothalamic gliomas (bulky lesions).
- *Presentation:*
  - *Optic nerve tumors:* Asymptomatic, long-standing proptosis, impaired visual acuity, optic nerve atrophy
  - *Chiasmal tumors:* Decreased visual acuity, temporal field defects chiasmatic
  - *Hypothalamic tumors:* Nystagmus, visual field deficits, impaired visual acuity, hydrocephalus, increased intracranial pressure.
- *On MRI:* Small and well-circumscribed, homogeneous enhancement.
- *Treatment:*
  - *Optic nerve and chiasmatic tumors:* Chemotherapy first for all patients and reserve RT for chemotherapy failures.
  - *Hypothalamic tumors:* CSF diversion if indicated. Maximal safe surgical resection, chemotherapy.
  - Radiotherapy is reserved (45–50 Gy) for patients who progress on or after chemotherapy.

CNS Lymphoma

High dose chemotherapy (IV/IT MTX, Vincristine, Procarbazine based). Corticosteroids should be avoided until MRI and biopsy due to its antitumor effect and repair of blood brain barrier which may decrease the delivery of drugs into brain parenchyma.

EBRT: Whole brain RT- 45 Gy in 25 fractions if no chemotherapy.
23.4 Gy in 1.8 Gy fractions if chemotherapy

Ependymoma

For negative CSF cytology:
GTR/STR → Limited field radiotherapy 54–60 Gy.
For positive CSF cytology:
GTR/STR → Craniospinal irradiation 36 Gy, boost to gross disease up to 54–60 Gy.

Choroid Plexus Tumors

- *Papilloma:* 60–80% (WHO Grade-I)
- *Carcinoma:* 20–40% (WHO Grade-III)

Treatment Recommendation

Choroid Plexus Papilloma

- *GTR and CSF negative*: Observation.
- *STR and CSF negative*: Radiotherapy to postoperative bed 50–54 Gy.
- *STR and CSF positive*: Craniospinal radiotherapy 36 Gy + limited field boost radiotherapy 54 Gy.

Choroid Plexus Carcinoma

- *GTR and CSF negative*: Radiotherapy 50 Gy
- *STR and CSF negative*: Radiotherapy to postoperative bed 54 Gy.
- *STR and CSF positive*: Craniospinal radiotherapy 36 Gy + limited field boost radiotherapy 54 Gy.

Meningioma

- *Operable:* Preoperative angiography for embolization → GTR → Observation with serial MRI → Radiotherapy in recurrence cases.

- *Inoperable:* Definitive radiotherapy or SRS.
- *Recurrence:* Radiotherapy or SRS as salvage therapy.

Doses: 54 Gy for benign, 60 Gy for malignant tumors.

SRS: Dose chosen based on tumor volume, location, surgical history, and radiosensitivity of critical organs.

Acoustic Neuroma

Surgery: Total or near total resection.
- If subtotal resection; postoperative radiotherapy is recommended.
- Preservation of cranial nerve VII >60%.
- Preservation of useful hearing 30–50%.

SRS: 12–13 Gy single fraction.
- Preservation of cranial nerve VII >90%
- Preservation of useful hearing—75%
- Preservation of cranial nerve V—>90%

Radical radiotherapy: 54 Gy in 28#.
- Preservation of cranial nerve VII — >95%
- Preservation of useful hearing — 75%
- Preservation of cranial nerve V — >95%

Pituitary tumors
Craniopharyngioma
Pineal tumors   Discussed in Pediatric Oncology
Germinomas   Chapter
Medulloblastoma

Primary Spinal Cord Tumors

- 2/3 extramedullary
- 1/3 intramedullary.

Intramedullary

- Astrocytoma (most common)
- Ependymoma
- Oligodendroglioma.

Intradural

Extramedullary:
- Meningioma
- Ependymomas
- Nerve sheath tumor.

Extradural

Metastasis, osteogenic osteosarcoma, chondrosarcoma, chondroma, myeloma, epidural hemangiomas, lipomas, meningioma and lymphomas.

Astrocytomas are most common in cervicothoracic spine.

Ependymomas are most common in LS spine.

Treatment:
- *All tumors resectable:* Maximal safe resection
- *Low-grade glioma:* Gross total resection → Observation
- *Low-grade glioma:* Subtotal resection → Radiotherapy 50–54 Gy
- *High-grade glioma:* 54 Gy
- *Ependymoma:* Radiotherapy to 50–54 Gy ± CSI
- *Meningioma, GTR:* Observation
- *Meningioma, STR:* RT 50–54 Gy.

Spinal cord sarcomas, vertebral bodies chondromas, chondrosarcomas and osteogenic sarcomas ⎤ SRT/Charged particle therapy

Arteriovenous Malformation

- *Resection:* Microsurgical or SRS.
  Entire nidus is treated but not feeding arteries or draining vessels.
- *Dose:* 21 Gy when treated with SRS.

Trigeminal Neuralgia

Medical Management

Carbamazepine, gabapentin, antidepressants, etc.

Surgical Options

Nerve blocks, partial sensory rhizotomy, balloon decompression of gasserian ganglion, microvascular decompression and peripheral nerve ablation.
Dose: SRS may also be used. 80 Gy.

FOLLOW-UP PROTOCOL

- 1st follow-up 6 weeks after completion of treatment (CT/MRI to be done at 2nd follow-up).
- Subsequent follow-up at 2 monthly intervals in 1st year.
- From 2nd year onwards, follow-up at 3 monthly intervals.

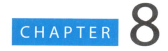

CHAPTER 8

Central Nervous System Tumors in Children

Ashutosh Mukherji

Radiotherapy for pediatric malignancies differs from adult treatment in three fundamental aspects:

1. Many pediatric tumors are radio-responsive and require relatively low doses, especially as chemotherapy is also used.
2. Growing tissues in children are likely to suffer more damage from radiotherapy than their adult counterparts and radiotherapy may sometimes have to be delayed.
3. Immobilization of young children is a major issue, not seen in adult patients. Target volumes are generally well-defined, with narrow margins, and hence immobilization is necessary. Children below 4–5 years of age may require anesthesia.

The CNS tumors are the most common solid tumors in childhood, accounting for 20–25% of all malignances. Most commonly include:

1. Neuroepithelial tumors
   - Astrocytomas
   - Ependymomas
   - Choroid plexus tumors
   - Neuronal and mixed glial tumors
   - Pineal parenchymal tumors
   - Embryonal tumors
2. Tumors of the meninges
3. Lymphomas and hematogenous malignancies
4. Germ cell tumors
5. Tumors of sellar region

ASTROCYTOMAS

Low-grade Astrocytomas

Surgery is the mainstay of treatment, with 80% of cerebral, cerebellar and spinal cord tumors; and 40% of diencephalic tumors amenable for complete surgical resection.

Indications for Radiotherapy

- Following incomplete resection in areas where tumor progression would compromise neurological functions.
- Patients with progressive and/or symptomatic disease that is unresectable.
  Radiotherapy is otherwise not indicated after complete resection.

Radiotherapy Target Volume

- *GTV:* It is the enhancement seen in the initial imaging study or at simulation, and is the region of enhancement on a T1 MRI sequence with gadolinium enhancement (or as seen on a T2 or flair sequence for non-enhancing lesions).
- *CTV:* For pilocytic astrocytomas includes GTV contoured on T1 MRI film plus 0.5 cm; while for fibrillary astrocytomas includes GTV on T2 (FLAIR) films plus 1–1.5 cm margin.
- *PTV:* CTV plus 0.3–0.5 cm if perspex mask is used; and margin of 0.1–0.2 cm if rigid/stereotactic frame is used.

Radiotherapy Dose

- *Postoperative radiotherapy:* The general trend is to deliver at least 45 Gy to all brain at risk (wide-field irradiation), followed by a field cone down to a more conformal boost volume.

  For children between the ages of 2 and 5 years, typical doses are 50 to 54 Gy in 150 to 180 cGy fractions. Radiation should be delayed, if possible, for children under the age of 2 years.

For children older than 5 years of age, the standard dose of 54 Gy/30# is recommended.

- *Non-operated cases*: The dose is 54 Gy/30 #/6 weeks @180 cGy per fraction.

High-grade Astrocytomas

Include anaplastic astrocytomas as well as glioblastomas. Goal of surgery is maximal possible resection with good neurological outcome.

Indications for Radiotherapy

Postoperative radiotherapy is indicated in all cases of high-grade gliomas.

Radiotherapy Target Volume

- *GTV:* It is the enhancement seen in the initial imaging study or at simulation, and is the region of enhancement on a T1 MRI sequence with gadolinium enhancement (or as seen on a T2 or flair sequence for nonenhancing lesions). For grade IV astrocytoma (glioblastoma multiforme), GTV is the T1-enhancing abnormality on MRI. If there is no postoperative residual enhancement, the tumor resection cavity is defined as the GTV for purposes of treatment planning. The surrounding edema is not considered part of the GTV.
- *CTV1*: GTV plus 2–3 cm as initial therapy.
- *CTV2*: GTV plus 1–1.5 cm as boost volume.
- *PTV*: CTV plus 1–1.5 cm.

Radiotherapy Dose

- *Postoperative radiotherapy*: The general trend is to deliver at least 54 Gy to CTV1, followed by a field cone down to a more conformal boost volume (CTV2) and treating up to a total dose of 60 Gy.

- *Nonoperated cases*: The dose is 65 Gy/35 #/7 weeks @180 cGy per fraction.

Optic Nerve/Chiasmatic/Hypothalamic Gliomas

Surgery is the treatment of choice in localized disease. Chemotherapy is indicated in most cases as adjuvant treatment. Radiotherapy is highly effective at halting progression.

Indications for Radiotherapy

- Progressive disease on chemotherapy in children older than 10 years.
- Progressive disease at diagnosis or after surgery for older patients.

Radiotherapy Target Volume

- *GTV*: It is the enhancement seen in the initial imaging study or at simulation, and is the region of enhancement on a T1 MRI sequence with gadolinium enhancement (or as seen on a T2 or flair sequence for nonenhancing lesions).
- *CTV*: GTV plus 1–1.5 cm.
- *PTV*: CTV plus 1–1.5 cm.

Radiotherapy Dose

In younger children, local fields are treated to a dose of 50 Gy in fraction size of 180 cGy; while children older than 5 years of age are treated to a dose of 54 Gy/30 #/6 weeks.

Brainstem Gliomas

These are usually deeply infiltrative and seldom curable. These can also be either focal tumors (described as circumscribed lesions smaller than 2 cm on MRI); or as diffuse infiltrating lesions.

Surgery is treatment of choice for focal lesions or those that are surgically accessible.

Indications for Radiotherapy

- Rare patients with high grade gliomas.
- Patients with low grade gliomas found to have progressive disease in the early postoperative period.
- Surgically inaccessible tumors.
- Diffusely infiltrating gliomas of the pons.

Radiotherapy Target Volume

Similar to low grade gliomas. Target delineated by contrast enhanced MRI.

- *GTV:* It is the enhancement seen on a T1 MRI sequence with gadolinium enhancement in focal lesions or as seen on a T2 or flair sequence for non-enhancing diffuse infiltrating lesions.
- *CTV:* GTV plus 0.5–1 cm in focal and 1.5 cm in diffuse infiltrating lesions.
- *PTV:* CTV plus 1–1.5 cm.

Radiotherapy Dose

54 Gy/30 #/6 weeks @180 cGy per fraction.

Astrocytomas of Spinal Cord

In the past, these were usually treated by biopsy followed by radiotherapy. Complete or subtotal resection is now possible in over 80% of cases. Chemotherapy may be an alternative in very young children and infants to delay radiotherapy.

Indications for Radiotherapy

- Patients with high grade gliomas.
- Older children with low grade gliomas found to have progressive disease in the early postoperative period.

- Surgically inaccessible tumors.
- Diffusely infiltrating/high grade gliomas.

Radiotherapy Target Volume

Target delineated by contrast enhanced MRI.
- *GTV:* Includes solid portion of the tumor including intra-tumoral cysts.
- *CTV:* GTV plus 0.5–1 cm in low grade lesions and 1.5 cm in high grade lesions.
- *PTV:* CTV plus 1–1.5 cm.

Radiotherapy Dose

50.4 Gy/28 #/5.3 weeks @180 cGy per fraction.

Mixed Neuronal-glial Tumors

These include gangliogliomas, anaplastic gangliogliomas and central neurocytomas. Surgery is treatment of choice.

Indication for Radiotherapy

- Sub-totally resected tumor.
- Progression/Recurrence after total excision.
- Atypical histology.
- MIB-1 labeling index > 3%.

Dose

54 Gy/30 #/6 weeks @180 cGy per fraction by two parallel opposed fields with 6 MV photons.

Radiotherapy Target Volume

- *GTV:* It includes the whole tumor based on preoperative imaging and any macroscopic residual disease.

- *CTV*: GTV plus 1 cm.
- *PTV*: CTV plus 0.5 cm.

EPENDYMOMAS

These have a predilection for infants and children younger than 5 years age. Spread through foramen magnum inferiorly is not uncommon. Gadolinium enhanced MRI of the entire craniospinal axis and CSF cytology are a pre-requisite for treatment planning.

Indication for Radiotherapy

Postoperative radiotherapy is indicated in all cases. Radiotherapy can be avoided in only the following situations:

a. Ependymoma of spinal cord post complete resection, and
b. In selected supra-tentorial ependymomas involving non-eloquent areas and are resected with wide margins.

Local RT is now the standard of care. Craniospinal irradiation (CSI) is only indicated in anaplastic ependymoma in presence of leptomeningeal seedings.

Radiotherapy Target Volume

- *GTV*: It includes tumor based on preoperative imaging and any macroscopic residual disease.
- *CTV*: GTV plus 1 cm in ependymomas and 1.5 cm in anaplastic as well as myxopapillary ependymomas.
- *PTV*: CTV plus 1-1.5 cm.

Radiotherapy Dose

54 Gy/30 #/6 weeks @180 cGy per fraction for ependymomas. In case of anaplastic ependymomas, 54 Gy/30 #/6 wk followed by a boost to macroscopic residual disease to a dose of 59–60 Gy. If leptomeningeal seedings are present, CSI of 36 Gy/20# followed by posterior fossa boost to 54 Gy is given. In case of myxopapillary

ependymomas, dose of 50.4 Gy is prescribed. CSI is given in case of leptomeningeal seedings.

CHOROID PLEXUS TUMORS

Surgery is the treatment of choice. Chemotherapy is given in young children to delay postoperative radiotherapy.

Indications for Radiotherapy

- Atypical tumors.
- Leptomeningeal seedings. CSI to be given.
- Postoperative residual disease.

Dose

54 Gy/30 #/6 weeks @ 180 cGy per fraction. If leptomeningeal seedings are present, CSI of 36 Gy/20# followed by posterior fossa boost to 54 Gy is given.

Radiotherapy Target Volume

- *GTV:* It includes tumor based on preoperative imaging and any macroscopic residual disease.
- *CTV:* GTV plus 1 cm in papillomas and 1.5 cm in atypical tumors.
- *PTV:* CTV plus 1–1.5 cm.

CRANIOPHARYNGIOMAS/SELLAR TUMORS

Craniopharyngiomas are among the most common suprasellar tumors in children and young adults. Surgery is treatment of choice.

Indications for Radiotherapy

- Subtotally resected tumor.
- Recurrence after total excision.

Dose

54 Gy/30 #/6 weeks @180 cGy per fraction by two parallel opposed fields with 6 MV photons for craniopharyngiomas; 50.4 Gy/28 #/6 weeks for other sellar tumors.

Radiotherapy Target Volume

- *GTV:* It includes the whole tumor (solid plus cystic areas) based on preoperative imaging and any macroscopic residual disease.
- *CTV*: GTV plus 1 cm.
- *PTV:* CTV plus 0.5 cm.

PINEAL TUMORS

Includes pinealoblastomas, pinealocytomas and intermediate grade tumors.

Indication for Radiotherapy

- Sub-totally resected tumor.
- Leptomeningeal seedings.

Dose

54 Gy/30 #/6 weeks @180 cGy per fraction with standard CSI of 36 Gy followed by local boost.

Radiotherapy Target Volume

- *GTV:* It includes the whole tumor (solid plus cystic areas) based on preoperative imaging and any macroscopic residual disease.
- *CTV:* Margin of 1–1.5 cm.

Whole ventricle therapy may be used.

MEDULLOBLASTOMAS

It is a radio-responsive and chemo-responsive tumor that arises in the cerebellum and has all the histologic characteristics of a PNET.

It is currently staged as high-risk and low-risk. High-risk cases include those with more than 1.5 cm^3 of residual tumor postoperatively, age below 3 years, high-grade histology, or metastatic disease anywhere in the craniospinal axis (cerebrospinal fluid [CSF] or gross disease). Surgery is necessary, with posterior midline craniotomy and attempted total excision being done. Radiotherapy is required in all cases.

Dose

Standard Risk Cases

(A) Standard dose CSI of 36 Gy/20 #/4 weeks followed by posterior fossa boost to a dose of 19.8 Gy/11 #/2.2 weeks by 2 parallel opposed fields.

(B) Low CSI dose schedule 23.4 Gy CSI @1800 Gy/# with concurrent vincristine chemotherapy followed by posterior fossa boost to total dose of 55.8 Gy/31#.

High-risk Cases

Standard dose CSI of 36 Gy/20 #/4 weeks followed by posterior fossa boost to a dose of 19.8 Gy/11 #/2.2 weeks by 2 parallel opposed fields. In case of leptomeningeal seedings, a 5–10 Gy boost may be given to whole spine after CSI. This is followed by 6 cycles of chemotherapy with either ICE or PCV regime.

Radiotherapy Target Volume

- *GTV:* It includes tumor based on preoperative imaging and any macroscopic residual disease. CT simulation is done for treatment planning. MRI is done to image lower extent of cord.
- *CTV:* It includes whole brain and spine till S3. Laterally includes nerve roots from intervertebral foramina. Cranial field is till C2-3. Spinal fields divided lengthwise into 2 fields.
- *PTV:* CTV plus 1 cm.

SUPRATENTORIAL PRIMITIVE NEUROECTODERMAL TUMORS

This is an aggressive infiltrative neoplasm that spreads widely throughout the CNS and carries a poor prognosis despite aggressive CSI. Maximal surgical excision is done. Postoperative radiotherapy is indicated in all cases followed by chemotherapy.

Radiation Dose

As for high-risk medulloblastoma.

GERM CELL TUMORS

Differentiated into germinomas and non-germinomatous GCTs.

Indication for Radiotherapy

All cases, especially germinomas.

Dose

Germinomas

Standard CSI to a dose of 30 Gy/20 #/4 weeks @ 150 cGy per fraction followed by a boost of 15 Gy/10 #/2 weeks to total dose of 45 Gy/30 #/6 weeks.

Nongerminomatous GCTs

54 Gy/30 #/6 weeks @ 180 cGy per fraction with standard CSI of 36 Gy followed by local boost up to 54 Gy.

Radiotherapy Target Volume

- *GTV:* It includes the whole tumor (solid plus cystic areas) based on preoperative and prechemotherapy imaging and any macroscopic residual disease.
- *CTV:* GTV plus margin of 1–1.5 cm.

Whole ventricle therapy may be used.

RADIOTHERAPY TECHNIQUE (BRAIN TUMORS)

For larger lesions, such as diffuse gliomas outside the brainstem, opposed lateral fields may provide appropriate coverage. When the PTV can be made smaller, a three-field technique using wedges can provide a highly conformal dose distribution. IMRT can further improve the dose conformity, but the increase in treatment time may be counterproductive with pediatric patients if anesthesia is also being used. SRT generally uses a hypofractionated treatment schedule, which may be highly preferred for children.

Patient Positioning

The head, neck, and body should be positioned such that the anterior and lateral setup marks are in locatable and reproducible positions. A neutral head position with the patient supine is easily reproducible and can be used in most situations, with the exception of posteriorly located tumors and craniospinal axis irradiation or other treatment involving the spinal cord. CT scan simulation, 3-D treatment planning and IMRT allow for neutral head and neck position in most situations as noncoplanar beams can be used to avoid entry and exit dose to organs at risk (OAR).

Immobilization

Variability of set-up should be not more than 2–3 mm with a thermoplastic mask. More accurate and/or rigid head positioning and immobilization can be obtained by a modified stereotactic head frame with noninvasive multiple-point head fixation.

After the patient is placed in the positioning device, they are scanned, with radiopaque reference markers placed at the setup isocenter. The isocenter may be placed at a standard location on every patient with a planned isocenter shift taking place after simulation. Verification films should be taken before treatment; these should include orthogonal radiographs to verify the isocenter, and films of any custom-shaped portal fields.

Simulation

For CT scan simulation involving the brain, the patient is placed in the positioning device and scanned with three radio-opaque reference markers placed on the thermoplastic mask. A prone setup may be considered for posterior fossa tumors. For intracranial disease, a single-field or opposed-beam two-field arrangements are usually not favored, as they deliver excessive dose to normal tissues in the beam paths. The exception is a short course of palliative radiation therapy to the whole brain or cervical spinal cord using an opposed lateral beam arrangement. An optimum beam arrangement typically consists of 3 to 7 nonopposed shaped beams. When applicable, the contralateral uninvolved hemisphere of the brain should be spared as much as possible. A true vertex beam should be avoided, if possible, due to exit dose into the body; a 5–10° Gantry rotation should be considered instead.

Beams

Most lesions can be treated well with 4–6 MV photons; for some deeper seated targets, 10-MV photons may provide slightly better dose distribution with respect to normal tissues, although with small targets penumbra issues may dominate. For lateralized tumors, 10-MV photons or differential weighting of beams may be used for the contralateral beam.

In case of infratentorial tumors, the posterior fossa must be boosted, with the anterior border covering the posterior clinoids and the superior border including 1 cm above halfway between the foramen magnum and vertex (superior extent to tentorium cerebelli). Inferiorly, the field should cover the foramen magnum.

Whole Brain Irradiation

Most often accomplished with opposed lateral fields. The patient is treated supine unless the spine is also to be treated. The field size is set to encompass the whole brain, with german helmet technique to exclude the anterior part of the eyes. The optic nerve and also the (cribriform plate) are sites for relapse and must be included. Setting the center of the field to the posterior orbit and blocking to protect the anterior portion of the orbit also eliminates beam divergence to the opposite eye. The radiation beam energy usually employed is 6-MV X-rays, although 4-MV or cobalt teletherapy may be used as effectively for most children. Lens dose can be reduced by placing the central axis at the lateral orbital rim to eliminate beam divergence or by rotating the beam posteriorly approximately 5°.

Intensity-Modulated Radiation Therapy

Intensity-Modulated Radiation Therapy (IMRT) may be used to improve dose delivery to target volumes which can reduce dose to the many dose-limiting OARs within the cranium, including the optic chiasm, right and left optic nerves, both globes, the brainstem, the right and left inner ear, the area postrema, and uninvolved normal brain, especially optic cortex and right and left temporal lobes. Reducing dose to the area postrema may reduce the incidence of treatment-related nausea. IMRT in craniospinal axis irradiation, can homogenize dose and improve conformality.

Craniospinal Irradiation

When the entire craniospinal axis is to be irradiated, the patient is usually simulated in the prone position with careful attention to immobilization technique and reproducibility. For the posterior fossa boost, the standard supine position is usually used, sometimes with extension of the neck to allow for posterior beams that do not exit through the eyes. OARs to be contoured include the brainstem, temporal lobes, and middle and inner ear regions. Decreasing the radiation dose delivered to the cochlea and eighth cranial nerve (auditory apparatus) in pediatric patients treated for medulloblastomas significantly reduces the risk of hearing loss.

Minimizing cochlear doses, particularly in patients receiving potentially ototoxic chemotherapy is therefore recommended for patients receiving posterior fossa irradiation. Therefore, true opposed-lateral beams should not be used; instead, two opposed beams should be angled anteriorly. The radiation beam energy usually employed is 6-MV X-rays, although 4-MV or cobalt teletherapy is as effective for most children. Lens dose can be reduced by placing the central axis at the lateral orbital rim to eliminate beam divergence or by rotating the beam posteriorly approximately 5°.

The intracranial area and upper one or two segments of the cervical cord are treated through two opposed lateral fields, positioned so that the isocenter is at midline with the beam axes passing through the lateral canthi to minimize divergence into the contralateral eye. Customized blocks protect the normal head and neck tissues from the primary radiation beam. Care must be taken not to underdose the cribriform plate. The inferior border of the initial cranial field is placed around C2-3, leaving adequate room for subsequent shifts in the match with the upper spine field. Depending on length, the spine is treated through one or two posterior fields. Usually field length of upper spinal field is maximized (40 cm at 100 cm SSD) and lower field is minimized to plan for junction shifts. If 40 cm or less of length covers the spine till the end of the thecal sac (near the level of S3), a lower spine field is not necessary. The caudal border of the lower PA spine field should be set inferior to S3 by a length equal to the two-field shifts, and then blocked back to S3 using asymmetric collimators or custom blocking.

Matching the upper border of the spine field to the lower border of the cranial field requires strict attention to accuracy, as overlap in the upper cervical cord may have serious sequelae. In one method, the collimator for the lateral cranial fields is angled to match the divergence of the upper border of the adjacent spinal field, and

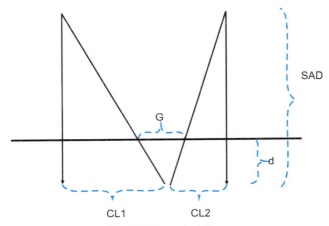

Fig. 8.1 Gap calculation

the treatment couch is angled so that the inferior border of the cranial field is perpendicular to the superior edge of the spinal field. The drawback to this technique is that the couch rotation displaces the contralateral eye superiorly, so that it cannot be blocked without blocking frontal brain tissue. This technique may also result in underdosing of the temporal lobes and cribriform plate. Alternatively, skin gaps are calculated appropriately (the collimator should still be rotated for accurate alignment) **(Fig. 8.1)**. The gap is calculated so that the 50% isodose lines meet at the level of the anterior spinal cord.

All junction lines are moved 0.5 to 1.0 cm every 8 to 12 Gy to avoid overdosing or under dosing segments of the cord. This is accomplished by shortening the inferior margin of the lateral cranial fields, symmetrically lengthening the superior and inferior margins of the posterior spine field, and shortening the cranial margin of the caudal spinal field.

Formula for gap correction in craniospinal RT

$$G = \frac{(CL1 + CL2) \times d}{SAD}$$

Where   G stands for gap to be calculated

CL is the field length from isocenter to the field edge to be matched

d is the depth at the match point

and   SAD is the source-axis distance.

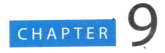

CHAPTER 9

Non-CNS Solid Tumors in Children

Ashutosh Mukherji

These include various other tumors apart from the CNS malignancies involving various systems.

RETINOBLASTOMA

Are 60–70% unilateral and are nearly always detected in the first 3 years of life. Patients are usually cured, and enucleation is recommended for eyes that have little potential for useful vision, especially in most unilateral disease and frequently the worse (blind) eye in bilateral retinoblastoma. Modalities of treatment include surgery (Enucleation), photocoagulation, cryotherapy, radiotherapy and use of radioactive plaques.

Treatment

Work-up

1. Histopathology includes external ocular examination, slit-lamp bimicroscopy, and biocular indirect ophthalmoscopy (under anesthesia for mapping).
2. *Laboratories:* CBC, chemistries, BUN, Cr, LFTs.
3. *Imaging:* Fluorescein angiography, bilateral USG (A and B mode) and MRI.
4. Bone scan and/or lumbar puncture for symptoms or suspected metastatic disease.
5. Risk factors for metastatic disease include optic nerve invasion, uveal invasion, orbital invasion, and choroidal involvement.

Stage and Treatment Recommendation

Unilateral intraocular

- Laser therapy with or without chemo-reduction × 6 cycles →
  focal therapy. Chemo-agents include vincristine, carboplatin,
  and etoposide. Focal therapy options include: EBRT (35–46
  Gy) for small tumors located within macula, diffuse vitreous
  seeding, or multifocal tumors.
- Cryotherapy is used in addition to EBRT or in place of
  photocoagulation for lesions <4 disc diameter (DD) in the
  anterior retina.
- Photocoagulation is used for posteriorly located tumors <4
  DD distinct from the optic nerve head and macula. It may be
  occasionally used alone for small tumors, or in addition to
  EBRT.
- Episcleral plaque brachytherapy is used for either focal
  unilateral disease or recurrent disease following prior EBRT.
- Enucleation if the tumor is massive or if the eye is unlikely to
  have useful vision after treatment.

Bilateral

- Each eye is assessed individually.
- The worse eye may or may not be enucleated depending on
  symptoms.
- If there is potential vision preservation in both eyes, bilateral
  chemo-reduction ± EBRT with close follow-up for focal
  treatment may be used.

Extraocular: Orbital EBRT + chemotherapy for palliation. High-dose
chemotherapy with stem cell rescue may be given in select cases.
Intrathecal chemotherapy may be given for patients with CNS or
meningeal disease.

Trilateral retinoblastoma: Neurosurgical resection, chemotherapy,
with cranial RT or CSI. Eyes are treated as per above mentioned
recommendations.

Indications for Radiotherapy

Brachytherapy

- For small tumors (2- to 3-disc diameter).
- Solitary lesions.
- Located more than 3 mm from optic disc.
- Tumor less than 10 mm thick.
- Choroidal extension of tumor.

Teletherapy

- To preserve vision.
- Lesions close to macula/optic nerve.
- Large lesions with vitreous seeding.
- Recurrent disease.
- Multifocal lesions.
- Adjuvant therapy after enucleation/evisceration.
- Palliative radiotherapy.

Radiotherapy Target Volume

The entire retina is treated including 5–8 mm of proximal optic nerve. The tumor is treated to a 98% isodose, while the rest of the orbital structures are encompassed in 50% isodose line.

Critical structures: Opposite eye, chiasma, pituitary gland, brainstem, posterior most teeth and upper cervical spine.

- *Group I and II lesions (close to macula/optic nerve):*
  - When optic nerve is involved:
    CTV: Entire retina up to ora serrata.
    PTV: CTV plus 5 mm.
  - When optic nerve is free:
    CTV: Proximal 1 cm of optic nerve.
    PTV: CTV plus 5 mm.

- *Group III, IV and V lesions:*
  - When optic nerve is involved:
    CTV: Entire retina up to ora serrata.
    PTV: CTV plus 5 mm.
  - When optic nerve is free:
    CTV: Proximal 1 cm of optic nerve.
    PTV: CTV plus 5 mm.
- *Postoperative (in locally advanced lesions):*
  Target volume includes entire orbit (GTV) + 5 mm (PTV). Any other disease extension is to be covered as well.

Radiotherapy Dose

- *Dose for Group I and II lesions:* 45 Gy/25 # /5 weeks for daily treatment; *or* 45 Gy/18 # /6 weeks @ 2.5 Gy per fraction alternate day treatment.
- *Dose for Group III, IV and V lesions:* 50.4 Gy / 28 # / 6 weeks for daily treatment; *or* 50.4 Gy / 20 # /7 weeks @ 2.5 Gy per fraction alternate day treatment.
- *Dose for postoperative microscopic residual lesions:* 45 Gy/25 # /5 weeks for daily treatment; *or* 45 Gy/18 # /6 weeks @ 2.5 Gy per fraction alternate day treatment.
- *Dose for postoperative gross residual lesions:* 50.4 Gy/28 # /6 weeks for daily treatment; *or* 50.4 Gy/20 # /7 weeks @ 2.5 Gy per fraction alternate day treatment.
- *Children below 1 year age:*
  Microscopic disease (postoperative) – 39.6 Gy/22 # /4.5 weeks.
  Gross disease – 45 Gy/25 # /5 weeks.
- *Brachytherapy:* 40 Gy to apex and 100–150 Gy to sclera (base of tumor).
- *Intracranial extension:* WBRT of 25 Gy/15 # @ 1.8 gy per fraction plus primary tumor treatment.
- *Metastases:* 15 Gy/5 fractions or 5 Gy single fraction depending on site.

Radiation Technique

EBRT

- Indicated for small tumors involving macula, diffuse vitreous seeding, or multifocal tumors or those that failed prior chemotherapy and local therapy.
- Pediatric anesthesia may be required with patient being simulated supine with thermoplastic head mask immobilization.
- Conformal radiotherapy is recommended using CT and/or MRI based planning with 4–6 MV photons used.
- For unilateral RB, four anterior oblique noncoplanar fields may be used (superior, inferior, medial, and lateral).
- For bilateral RB when both eyes require treatment, 3DCRT (or IMRT) is used with opposed lateral fields and anterior oblique fields. Lateral fields may be angled 5 degree posteriorly to avoid exit dose to opposite eye.
- Depending on stage and anatomy, 0.5 cm bolus may be required.
- At a minimum, the entire retina is treated including 5–8 mm of the optic nerve.
- Dose delivered is 42–45 Gy in 1.8–2 Gy fractions and sometimes up to 50 Gy may be prescribed for larger tumors.
- Critical structures to limit RT dose include the opposite globe (including lens and retina), lacrimal glands, optic chiasma, pituitary gland, brainstem, posterior mandibular teeth, and upper cervical spine.

Episcleral Plaque Brachytherapy

- The treatment volume covers the tumor + radial margin of ~2 mm and deep margin of 1–2 mm.
- The dose to the tumor apex is 40 Gy, while the base receives 100–200 Gy.
- The dose rate is 0.7–1.0 Gy/h, and given over 2–4 days.

WILMS' TUMOR

It is highly responsive to both radiation as well as chemotherapy. Patients are divided into 3 risk groups: low, intermediate, and high (**Table 9.1**).

In the low-risk group, the chemotherapy consists of 18 weeks of actinomycin D and vincristine. For the intermediate group, doxorubicin is added to the chemotherapy regimen. In the high-risk group, etoposide is added, except for the rhabdoid tumors where

Table 9.1 National Wilms' tumor studies (NWTS)-5 risk categories and treatment strategies

Risk	Stage	Characteristics	Treatment
Low	I	Favorable histology, focal or diffuse anaplasia	Surgery + 18 wk chemo
	II	Favorable histology	Surgery + 18 wk chemo
Intermediate	III, IV	Favorable histology	Surgery + 24 wk chemo + RT (10 Gy to tumor bed + 12 Gy to lung mets)
	IIa - IV	Focal anaplasia	Surgery + 24 wk chemo + RT (10 Gy to tumor bed + 12 Gy to lung mets)
	IV	Favorable histology plus lung mets on computed tomography scan	Surgery + 24 wk chemo + RT (10 Gy to tumor bed + 12 Gy to lung mets)
High	IIa-IV	Diffuse anaplasia	Surgery + 24 wk chemo + RT (10 Gy to tumor bed + 12 Gy to lung mets)
	Ia-V	Clear cell renal tumors	Surgery + 24 wk chemo + RT (10 Gy to tumor bed + 12 Gy to lung mets)
	Ia-IV	Rhabdoid tumors	Surgery + 24 wk chemo (carboplatin, etoposide, and cyclophosphamide)

Abbreviations: RT, radiotherapy; Chemo, chemotherapy; wk, weeks

the chemotherapy is different. For certain patients with stage I and favorable histology, tumors will be treated with surgery alone.

Principles of Radiotherapy

- Should be started within 10 days of surgery.
- No change in dose for favorable or unfavorable type.
- Rhabdoid tumors are treated as a separate entity.

Indications for Radiotherapy

- Stage II unfavorable histology
- Stage III and IV favorable and unfavorable histology.
- Local recurrence.
- For intermediate-risk patients, lung RT for pulmonary metastasis is indicated only if they have not responded to chemotherapy after 9 weeks of postoperative treatment.
- For high-risk patients, lung RT is always indicated for pulmonary metastasis.
- Whole-abdominal RT is indicated for all stage III disease in case of diffuse spillage or peritoneal metastasis.

Indications for Whole Abdominal Radiotherapy

- Peritoneal seeding.
- Gross residual abdominal disease.
- Diffuse spillage of tumor at surgery.
- Preoperative intraperitoneal rupture.

Radiotherapy Volume and Technique

Radiotherapy (RT) is generally delivered with an AP/PA technique. Fields are generally limited to the operative bed, which consists of the kidney outline and any associated tumor with 2–3 cm margin. The superior border of the fields should extend to the diaphragmatic dome only if there is tumor present. Fields should overlap the entire vertebral body but exclude the other kidney unless there is bilateral involvement.

In whole-abdomen radiation; fields may extend from the diaphragmatic dome to the obturator foramen with the femoral head blocked. The dose to the uninvolved kidney should be kept below 15 Gy. However, as most patients receive only 10 Gy, this is often not a problem. Shielding can be done with a kidney block on the posterior field at the start of treatment and an anterior block added when organ tolerance is approached. Typical dose fractions can be as high as 2 Gy or as low as 1.5 Gy for large treatment volumes. When pulmonary metastases are present, bilateral lung irradiation can be given along with abdominal irradiation. Fields extend from the clavicles to approximately L1 with the shoulders appropriately blocked. Mediastinal blocks are never used.

Radiotherapy Dose

- Stage I and II FH; Stage I Anaplastic: No RT.
- Stage III FH, Stage I-III focal anaplasia, Stage I-II diffuse anaplasia, Stage I-III CCSK: Postoperative 10.8 Gy to flank and tumor bed plus 10 Gy boost to gross residual (>3 cm) disease.
- Stage III diffuse anaplasia, Stage I-III RTK: 19.8 Gy flank RT (10.8 Gy to infants).
- Stage IV (Lung Mets), FH: 12 Gy/8 # whole lung irradiation (WLI).
- Stage IV (Lung Mets), UFH: 12 Gy/8 # whole lung irradiation (WLI).
- Stage IV (Brain mets): 30.6 Gy/17 # WBRT or 21.6 Gy WBRT plus 10.8 Gy IMRT/SRT boost.
- Stage IV (Liver Mets): 19.8 Gy/11 # whole liver RT.
- Stage IV (Bone Mets): 25.2 Gy to tumor plus 3 cm margin.
- Unresected LN mets: 19.8 Gy.
- Relapsed abdominal disease: 12.6–18 Gy (in infants) and 21.6 Gy (older children) if previous radiation dose was less than 10.8 Gy. Boost dose of 9 Gy to gross residual disease after surgery.

NEUROBLASTOMA

The role of RT has diminished in recent years, as the good-prognosis tumors are often cured surgically and advanced disease usually indicates dissemination. But more than half of patients with neuroblastoma present with demonstrable metastases at diagnosis.

Indications for Radiotherapy

- Irradiation of positive regional lymph nodes.
- Total body irradiation: Preparatory regime for bone marrow transplant.
- Symptomatic in stage 4-S. The usual indication for RT is hepatomegaly causing respiratory compromise.
- Palliation.
- Iodine 131, metaiodobenzylguanidine (mIBG) avid on scan.
- Postoperative in high risk cases even after complete resection.

Radiotherapy Volume and Technique

For Abdominal Disease

- *GTV:* Volume of tumor before surgery and after induction chemotherapy as defined by CT or MRI.
- *CTV:* GTV plus a 1- to 2-cm margin. If spine is defined in the CTV, it is generally extended to include complete vertebral bodies to minimize differential growth effects.
- *PTV:* CTV plus 0.5 cm margin.

The dose objectives are:

a. Treat the entire CTV to 100% of the prescribed dose (about 20 Gy).
b. Keep one-third of the ipsilateral kidney below 16 Gy.
c. Keep two-thirds of the contralateral kidney below 16 Gy.
d. Doses to the liver, spleen, and stomach should be calculated and kept reasonable.
e. In stage 4-S, objective of the treatment is to reduce the size of the liver rather than to eliminate the tumor. The liver can be treated

with a single anterior field. However, lateral fields mainly avoid the right kidney and spine. Dose of 6 Gy/3 # is sufficient.

Radiotherapy Dose

Age <18 months:
Gross disease: 15 Gy (wide local field) + 10 Gy boost.
Microscopic disease: 15 Gy (wide local field) + 5 Gy boost.

Age > 19 months:
Gross disease: 20 Gy (wide local field) + 10 Gy boost.
Microscopic disease: 15 Gy (wide local field) + 10 Gy boost.

EWING'S SARCOMA

Prognosis for both local control and survival depends on the size of the tumor. Smaller tumors in expendable bones (e.g. fibula, ribs) can be cured by either surgery or RT, although surgery is often preferred. Larger tumors that are usually unresectable may require debulking surgery plus RT. Metastases remain the main cause for failure of treatment.

Indications for Radiotherapy

Preoperative Radiotherapy

• Avoid intralesional resection with comparable local control.

Postoperative Radiotherapy

• After intralesional or marginal resections.
• When a wide resection had poor histologic response (>10% residual tumor cells or <100% necrosis in the resected specimen).

Radiotherapy Volume and Technique

In all cases it is necessary to map the complete extent of disease using radiographs, T2-weighted MRI, and bone scans. Large soft tissue masses are initially treated with a 3-cm margin around the pre chemotherapy soft tissue tumor volume plus a 2-cm margin around the initial bony disease. In case of a complete response to chemotherapy, the margin is reduced to 1 cm around the original abnormality. RT may, under some circumstances, follow limb saving surgery when margins are suspect. Boost field includes the soft tissue component to the post-chemotherapy volume with a 2-cm margin. There is no field reduction for the bony disease.

Customized portals based on MRI planning are required for every case. A strip of normal tissue should be spared to ensure lymphatic drainage. Entire medullary cavity need not be irradiated.

Radiotherapy Dose

Preoperative Radiotherapy

Phase I: 45 Gy/25 # /5 weeks @ 180 cGy/#.

Phase II:
a. If there is complete response: No further boost.
b. Response to induction < 50%: 10.8 Gy/6 # /1 week @ 180 cGy/ #.
c. Response to induction > 50%: 14.4 Gy/8 # /1.5 weeks @ 180 cGy/#.
Surgery may be planned 6 weeks after RT.

Postoperative Radiotherapy

Phase I: 45 Gy/25 # / 5 weeks @ 180 cGy / #. No radiotherapy if negative margin and 100% necrosis.

Phase II:
a. If negative margin and <100% necrosis: No further boost.
b. If close margin and 100% necrosis: No further boost.
c. If close margin and <100% necrosis: 5.4 Gy/3 # /0.5 weeks @ 180 cGy/#.
d. If microscopic positive margin and 100% necrosis: No further boost.

e. If microscopic positive margin and <100% necrosis: 5.4 Gy/3 # /0.5 weeks @ 180 cGy/ #.

f. If gross positive margin and 100% necrosis: 5.4 Gy/3 # /0.5 weeks @ 180 cGy/ #.

g. If gross positive margin and <100% necrosis: 10.8 Gy/6 # /1 week @ 180 cGy/ #.

RHABDOMYOSARCOMA

Favorable sites are orbit, paratesticular, vagina, vulva, uterus, and superficial head and neck. Unfavorable sites are bladder, prostate, extremities, parameningeal head and neck, trunk, retroperitoneal, perineal, and perianal. IMRT and 3-DCRT are significantly better than conventional radiation therapy. Proton therapy allows the best dose conformality with minimal dose to surrounding critical structures.

Indications for Radiotherapy

To ensure adequate local control in cases unable to undergo complete wide surgical resection of tumor.

Radiotherapy Volume and Technique

- *GTV:* Extent of disease at diagnosis (pre-chemotherapy volume).
- *CTV:* GTV plus 1 cm.
- *PTV:* CTV plus 0.5 cm.

Margins depend upon site, immobilization, and image-guided verification techniques. Tight margins may be reasonable for head and neck therapy, but can be inappropriate for other sites.

Radiotherapy Dose

- In patients under 6 years old: 41.4 Gy for tumors <5 cm and 45 Gy for tumors 5 cm or more in greatest diameter.
- In patients 6 years or older: 45 Gy for <5 cm size lesions and 50.4 Gy for >5 cm lesions.

Fraction sizes of 180 cGy are used. Local control (LC) has been shown to be better for nonparameningeal head and neck RMS when doses >45 Gy are used. When tumor size exceeds 5 cm, LC improves for doses >47.5 Gy.

IRS-5 protocol has shown no loss of benefit in decreasing dose to 36 Gy in microscopic disease and to 45 Gy in group III orbital tumors.

CHILDHOOD LYMPHOMAS

Hodgkin's Disease

Primary chemotherapy, usually followed by involved-field RT to a dose of 15–25 Gy @ 1.5 Gy/fraction, is often preferred.

Involved-field RT in children requires precise staging and localization of involved nodes. Most treatments are done with an AP/PA technique. The most common site is the neck and supraclavicular nodes.

For children past the age of puberty, extended-field RT can be used as in an adult. For supra-diaphragmatic presentations this usually includes a tailored mantle field followed by a para-aortic field treated to the level of L4. For subdiaphragmatic presentation this usually includes para-aortic fields and inguino-iliac fields as an inverted Y.

Non-Hodgkin's Lymphomas

Indications for Radiotherapy

- Emergency radiotherapy for mediastinal masses and cranial nerve palsies.
- CNS irradiation in primary lymphomas or established CNS disease.
- Localized disease.
- Bone lymphoma (uncertain value).

- Transplantation (immunosuppression with total body irradiation). Techniques are tailored to each field and case.

LEUKEMIAS

Acute lymphoblastic leukemia (ALL) is the most common leukemia in children treated by the radiation oncologist.

Indications for Radiotherapy in ALL

- Prophylactic cranial irradiation (PCI).
- Treatment of central nervous system leukemia.
- Meningeal relapses.
- Testicular irradiation.
- Large mediastinal mass.
- Palliation.
- Total body irradiation (TBI) as preparation for bone marrow transplant.

Radiotherapy Doses

- *PCI:* 18 Gy in 10 fractions.
- *CNS leukemia:* 18–30 Gy in 1.8 Gy size fractions as CSI plus local boost with dose to spine not exceeding 15 Gy.
- *Testicular irradiation:* 24 Gy in 12 fractions as therapeutic and 12 Gy in 9 fractions as prophylactic.

Palliative: 2–6 Gy.

TBI: 12 Gy in 3–4 days.

Radiotherapy Volume and Technique

Therapeutic CNS irradiation: Technique described in CNS tumors for CSI. 6 MV photons preferred.

Prophylactic cranial irradiation (PCI): Treatment volume should include the subarachnoid space inside the vault. The inferior margin is the 2nd cervical vertebra and includes the whole vertebral body.

Treatment is generally given by two parallel opposed lateral fields. Special precaution is to be given to adequately cover the posterior part of globe, the cribriform plate and the middle cranial fossa while designing blocks for face (German Helmet technique). The anterior eye is protected by either using half-beam blocks and placing beam isocenter to just behind lens or by asking patients to look downwards. Beam energy of 6 MV photons is preferred so that dose build up is superficial to meninges.

Testicular irradiation: It is usually done with a single anteroposterior (AP) field set to the smallest field size. If a photon beam is used, it can be angled in the superior-inferior direction treating the testes tangentially. If an electron beam is used, it is setup en face to treat the testes directly. The penis is taped to the abdomen and out of the treatment field. The patient is placed in a frog-leg position. The scrotal sac may be taped in such a way so as to minimize the size of the electron cone needed. The testes should be centered in the field, and a bolus may be applied to bring the center of the testes to the depth of maximum dose. The field may be reduced as the testicular mass decreases in size during therapy. Electron energy is usually chosen to minimize dose beyond the target as much as possible.

Total body irradiation: Dose is prescribed to the midplane, usually at the level of the umbilicus. Compensators or bolus are used to maintain dose uniformity. Various techniques can be used like bilateral technique which has the advantage that the arms shield the heart and lungs; but the disadvantage is of a general need for bolus or specially designed compensators. An AP/PA technique is inherently simpler but often requires whole or partial blocks to shield the heart and lungs.

In general, higher-energy beams also improve dose uniformity but often require a bolus to increase skin dose. Lung blocking is typically employed lowering the midplane lung dose to 8 to 10 Gy. Computed tomography (CT) is useful for accurate lung dosimetry and block design. The dose-rate is kept under 10 cGy per minute to help reduce emesis, and hence large treatment rooms are generally required for larger patients and are an advantage even with smaller patients. Immobilization is important because treatment can last up to 40 minutes or more. Small children and infants require smaller fields and have relatively little variation in thickness throughout their anatomy and also often provide much less scatter than adults. Therefore, they can often be treated at an extended distance with a lower-energy beam. Infants can be treated on the floor with the gantry at zero degrees, underneath a spoiler that may also support lung blocks. The infant can be flipped from the supine to the prone position to allow an AP/PA treatment.

Total body irradiation (TBI) should always be set up as a special procedure with attention to the limitations of the room and equipment, as well as the nature of the patient. Most treatment planning systems do not permit treatment planning at the extended distances necessary for whole body irradiation. Individual patient dosimetry is important for monitoring the overall dose uniformity during treatment. Typically thermoluminescent dosimeters (TLDs) or diodes are used for the first or the first few treatments. Entrance and exit doses are measured at several points along the patient's anatomy.

HEPATOBLASTOMAS

Indication

- Preoperatively in unresectable disease after surgery.
- Postoperative residual disease.
- Palliative.

Radiation Dose

- *Limited volume:* 45 Gy for bulky disease and 35 Gy for microscopic disease.
- *Whole liver irradiation:* 20–25 Gy in 10–13 fractions.

Volume and Technique

Parallel opposed beams usually used. Multiple noncoplanar beams may also be used. 4–6 MV photons are preferred.

LANGERHANS CELL HISTIOCYTOSIS

Indication

- Local healing not achieved with surgery.
- Postoperative relapsed disease.
- *Palliative:* Nerve compression, pain relief.

Radiation Dose

- 10 Gy in conventional fractions.

CHAPTER 10

Genitourinary Cancer

Vikash Kumar, Ashutosh Mukherji

PROSTATE

Role of Radiotherapy

For stage I, II (T1 and T2N0) disease treatment options are:

- Radical surgery
- Radical radiotherapy or } Equally effective but morbidities vary.
- Wait and watch policy
- Radical interstitial brachytherapy (till T2a)
- Adjuvant hormonal ablation (bulky T2b onwards).

For stage III (T3N0):

- Radical radiotherapy
- Radical prostectomy
- Adjuvant hormonal ablation.

For stage IV (T4N1M1):

Palliative (Hormone ablation)

Indications of postoperative radiotherapy:

- Positive/close margins
- Positive lymph nodes
- Capsular invasion
- Seminal vesicle involvement
- Significant rise in PSA 3 weeks after surgery.
  Radiotherapy is postponed till 6 weeks after surgery to prevent stricture.

Five year survival after radiotherapy is 70–90% for T1/T2 disease and 50–70% for T3/T4 disease.

Conformal radiotherapy increases therapeutic ratio.

Neoadjuvant and concurrent androgen deprivation therapy has improved survival advantage.

Patients with enlarged pelvic nodes and metastatic disease (T4N1M1) are treated with primary hormone therapy.

Patients with disease confined to the prostate capsule (T1/T2a) can be treated by brachytherapy.

PLANNING TECHNIQUE

Assessment of Disease

- Digital rectal examination
- TRUS
- CT scan/MRI
- Bone scan (PSA > 20 n/mL, Gleason score 7 or more).

Definition of Target Volume

Gross tumor volume comprises the total prostate gland with base of the seminal vesicle; if seminal vesicle is grossly involved, the volume is extended posteriorly and superiorly.

Clinical target volume and planning tumor volume includes a margin of 1–1.5 cm inferiorly around prostate apex, superiorly above the apex of seminal vesicles, anteriorly towards the pubic symphysis and posteriorly, it includes 1 cm rectal wall.

Patient Positioning and Immobilization

Supine position with skin tattoos midline anteriorly over pubic symphysis and laterally over iliac crest to prevent lateral rotation and laser lights for accurate alignment.

Localization

Patient is asked to evacuate his bowel with comfortably full bladder with radiopaque markers over skin tattoos. CT scans are taken at 5 mm interval.

For 2D localization; the patient contour, target volume and the critical organs are marked in the CT slice taken from the center of the target volume. A margin of 1–1.5 cm is added to GTV assessed from serial images. If CT facility is not available; the tumor and critical organs are delineated by radiopaque contrast in bladder and rectum and an AP radiograph is taken.

For 3D localization; GTV, PTV and all critical organs are dilineated on each CT slice and a 3D reconstruction is produced.

FIELD ARRANGEMENTS

Either one anterior and two posterior oblique or one anterior and two parallel opposed lateral portals are usually preferred.

Posterior fields are wedged to compensate for patients contour and are angled at 120°.

Four-field box technique increases dose to posterior part and is beneficial when there is seminal vesicle involvement.

Implementation of Plan

Patient is treated in supine position; preferably with a high energy linac after rectal voiding and comfortably full bladder.

Alignment is done by matching orthogonal lasers with skin tattoos.

All fields are treated isocentrically (SAD technique).

Dose Prescription

50 Gy in 25 fractions over 5 weeks followed by 25 Gy boost (Total dose should be above 75 Gy for radical RT).

In postoperative cases; 46 Gy in 23 fractions to whole pelvis with 14 Gy boost.

Breast irradiation prior to antiandrogen therapy –15 Gy in 3 fractions over 3 days with 9–12 MeV electrons.

IMRT in Prostate Cancer

- Favorable group:
  T1, T2a
  Gleason score ≤ 6
  Low grade
  PSA <10

  Prostate only radiotherapy by 3D CRT or IMRT or brachytherapy (Dose: 72 Gy/40 fractions/8 weeks.) (76–80 Gy in conventional #)

- Unfavorable group:
  T2b, T2c, T3, T4
  Gleason score >6
  High grade
  PSA > 10

  46–70 Gy @ 2 Gy #
  Whole pelvic RT 4 field/3 field (45 Gy/25 Fr/5 weeks) followed by 3D CRT or IMRT or Brachytherapy (27 Gy/15 fractions/3 weeks)

BRACHYTHERAPY IN PROSTATE CANCER

Indications

- T1/T2 disease
- PSA < 20 ng/mL
- No prior prostate surgery
- Prostate volume <50 cc.
- Negative bone scan
- No pelvic lymphadenopathy

The preferred technique is TRUS and template guided implantation of iodine seeds via percutaneous route.

Volume of prostate, number and position of iodine seeds and template coordinates are determined by planning real time ultrasonography.

T1, T2a—HDR Monotherapy—48 Gy in 8 Fr over 1.5 week once daily.

T2b, T2c—HDR boost—6 Gy in 4 Fr, twice daily.

T3a-b—HDR boost—6 Gy in 4 Fr, twice daily.

RENAL CELL CARCINOMA

Role of Radiotherapy

- Adjuvant to surgical therapy
- Treatment of metastatic foci.

Indications of Postoperative Radiotherapy

- Perinephric fat involvement
- Rupture of fascia gerota
- Lymph node metastasis
- Vascular invasion.

(Postoperative radiotherapy should be delivered 4 weeks following surgery, a delay beyond 6 weeks causes development of resistant clones.)

Target Volume Includes

- Para-aortic nodes
- Hilar and perihilar lymph nodes
- Renal bed, and
- Surgical scar.

Field Arrangements

Parallel opposed AP-PA portals are used. Postoperative surgical clips at the operated site is the best guide for renal bed. Otherwise surface marking of kidney and draining lymph nodes with margins are used to dilineate field.

Dose Prescription

- *Postoperative*: 45–50 Gy in 5 weeks.
- *Palliative*: 30 Gy in 10 fractions over 2 weeks.

URINARY BLADDER CANCERS

Treatment of choice for superficial bladder tumors (of which the most common presentation is of Ta and T1 tumor) is TURBT especially for Ta, G1 tumors. High grade lesions may require adjuvant intravesical BCG. In muscle invasive bladder cancers radical cystectomy has been standard of care for two decades. But organ-preserving regimens using multiple-modality therapy, consisting of TUR followed by irradiation and concurrent chemotherapy, are emerging as viable alternatives. The ultimate goal is to maximize the quality of life by refining the treatment choice.

Radiation therapy for cancers of the urinary bladder can be delivered as external beam or as brachytherapy; and the intent of treatment can be:

- Preoperative
- Postoperative
- Concurrent chemoradiation as a part of multi-modality bladder sparing protocol
- Radiotherapy alone especially in elderly patients
- Palliative radiotherapy.

Indication for Radiotherapy

- **Definite setting/bladder preservation:**
    - Superficial tumor recurrence and/or progression after BCG instillation
    - Muscle-invading disease ($\geq$T2)
    - Patient refused radical cystectomy.
- **Adjuvant setting after radical cystectomy:**
    - Bladder has multiple tumors (>3) with at least one broad base tumor
    - Lymph node (+) or resection margin (+).
- **Palliative purpose:**
    - Unresectable disease
    - Painful disease or severe hematuria.

- **Preoperative radiotherapy:**
  - Tumor size reduction in locally advanced, muscle invasive disease, resulting in downstaging and make surgery easier
  - Decrease in the incidence of local recurrence following radical cystectomy
  - Decrease in the incidence of distant metastasis
  - Improvement of survival
  - No increase in the incidence of surgical complications.

Dose of Radiotherapy

- *Dose per fraction:* Once daliy 1.8–2 Gy; (Twice daily 1.5–1.6 Gy)
- *Total dose:*
  - 60–65 Gy to bladder tumor
  - 40–45 to pelvic lymph nodes
- *Normal tissue constraint*
  - *Rectum:*
    - i. V65 < 17%
    - ii. V40 < 35%
  - *Small bowel:*
    - i. Maximum dose < 5200 cGy
    - ii. Mean dose < 23.5 Gy
  - *Femoral head:* V50 < 5–10%

Target Volume

For external beam radiotherapy, initial treatment volume includes the whole bladder, proximal urethra, and in male patients, the prostate with the prostatic urethra and the regional lymphatics. The regional lymphatics adjacent to the bladder include hypogastric, external iliac, and obturator lymph nodes.

Common Definition of Radiation Portal of 4-field Technique

- Anteroposterior fields extend laterally 1.5 cm to the bony pelvis at its widest; exclude the inferior corners to protect femoral heads

- Lateral fields extend anteriorly 1.5–2 cm from the most anterior aspect of the bladder. The posterior border extends 2.5 cm posterior to the most posterior aspect of the bladder and falls within the rectum.
- *The inferior border*: Below the middle of the obturator foramen
- *The superior border*: L5-S1 or at the superior SI joint.
- A four-field box technique is used most frequently as it provides a relatively homogeneous dose distribution over the treated volume, while keeping the radiation dose outside this volume to about 50% of the intended tumor dose.
- Because much of the bladder is anterior to the coronal midplane, anterior weightage is given, relative to the posterior one.
- Boost volumes = entire bladder or partial bladder. CTV = GTV + 0.5–0.7 cm. PTV = CTV + 1.5 cm.

For IMRT Technique (Strongly Consider IGRT)
- *GTV*: Macroscopic tumor visible on CT/MRI/cystoscopy
- *CTV*: GTV + whole bladder + lymph nodes (obturator, external and internal iliac region) + proximal urethra + prostate + prostate urethra
- *PTV*: CTV + 1.5–2 and 2–3 cm superiorly (can probably be reduced to 1 cm and 1.5–2 cm superiorly with the use of fiducials + IGRT

Technique of Radiotherapy

- For treatment planning, a CT scan is performed with the patient supine in the treatment position with arms folded across the chest with ankle supports to stabilize the legs and pelvis, and a knee support for comfort.
- *For 2DRT:* The bladder should be emptied immediately before scanning and treatment, to reduce the volume irradiated and doses to normal tissues.
- *For 3DRT and IMRI:* Bladder protocols should be uniformly followed

- – In initial phase; a fixed time (20–30 minutes) after emptying bladder fixed amount of fluid (½–1 liter) should be given to partially distend bladder.
- – In phase 2, bladder is emptied before simulation and RT.
- The rectum should be empty to reduce organ motion and interfractional variations.
- A small volume of oral contrast is given 1 hour before the planning CT scan to show the small bowel.
- The scan is performed with 3–5 mm slices from the lower border of L5 to the inferior border of the ischial tuberosities.
- IMRT with inverse planning can reduce the dose to normal tissues, and allow the delivery of a synchronous boost needed for partial bladder irradiation and permit dose escalation to the tumor.
- However, IMRT for this tumor site requires excellent immobilization, with IGRT to locate and minimize PTV at the time of treatment. It has been shown that without IGRT an isotropic margin of 3 cm is required, but with IGRT this can be reduced to 12 mm.

Brachytherapy

- Interstitial therapy is not a common part of management of patients with bladder cancer.
- Brachytherapy for bladder cancer is limited almost exclusively to afterloaded interstitial therapy with iridium-192 (^{192}Ir) sources.
- A commonly accepted dimension of bladder tumors selected for brachytherapy is <5 cm.
- The tumor usually is treated with a single plane implant of three to five line sources: needles or catheters into which the radioactive sources will be loaded (30 Gy at 58 cGy per hour). The distance between line sources is about 1 cm. A single plane implant can be used to treat a 2–2.5 cm thick lesion; beyond that two-plane implants may become necessary.

Palliative Radiotherapy

- 21 Gy in 3 fractions given on alternate days in 1 week or 36 Gy in 6 fractions of 6 Gy given once weekly for 6 weeks.
- In most cases 21 Gy in 3 fractions on alternate days over 1 week is as effective as longer schedules for palliation as shown by the MRC BA09 trial.
- A weekly hypofractionated regimen of 6 Gy weekly for 6 fractions has been shown to effectively palliate symptoms in patients unfit for radical treatment and may be preferred by some patients.

Treatment Delivery and Patient Care

- Before radiation starts the patient should be made as fit as possible.
- Urinary infection should be treated, anemia should be corrected to hemoglobin 12 g/dL and a low residue diet advised.
- Radiation cystitis is common; infection should always be excluded and a high fluid intake advised.
- Catheterization should be avoided if possible to minimize the risk of infection.

Side Effects of Radiotherapy

- Acute complications mainly consist of bladder irritability, resulting from mucositis with decreased bladder capacity, which is manifested by frequency, urge incontinence, dysuria, diarrhea (usually mild) and anal irritation.
- Mild proctitis and lethargy are common.
- Late side effects include fibrosis and shrinkage of the bladder, hematuria due to bladder telangiectasia, late bowel damage, vaginal dryness and stenosis in women and impotence in men.

URETHRAL CANCERS

The main prognostic factors are tumor size and site, with better prognosis for distal locations. When the entire organ is involved, or when the tumor is fixed, infiltrating adjacent structures, or when there is lymph node metastasis, the prognosis is significantly worse. In locally extensive forms the best treatment may be surgery. For limited disease, according to the site of the tumor, brachytherapy has an important role, usually in combination with external beam irradiation or limited surgery, allowing a conservative approach. Lymph node involvement can be found in half of the patients.

Work-up and Investigations

- Clinical examination to determine if the tumor involves the urethral meatus and examination of the groin for palpable nodes.
- *General laboratory systematic studies:* Blood count and chemistry profile, urinary analysis.
- Further investigations are based on endoscopy and imaging. For primary lesions, the radiological examination of choice in the past used to be retrograde and antegrade urethrography. But now ultrasound, CT and MRI to allow precise definition of the tumor volume with associated local or locoregional extensions.
- Distant dissemination evaluated by chest radiograph, bone scan, liver CT, ultrasonography, as clinically indicated.
- While distant metastases are uncommon at the time of diagnosis, chest-radiograph is recommended.

Indication for Radiotherapy

Surgery

- Superficial lesions treated by intraluminal or laser resection.
- For locally extensive disease, radical surgery is indicated.

Radiotherapy

- The thickness of the tumor is not a definitive contraindication for brachytherapy as both intraluminal and interstitial therapy can be combined.
- Very bulky infiltrating tumors, particularly in female patients with lymph node involvement are treated with a combination of external beam irradiation to the primary tumor, groin and pelvic nodes plus brachytherapy boost to primary tumor.

Dose of Radiotherapy

- In case of LDR brachytherapy alone, the total dose is 60–65 Gy delivered in 3–5 days. The dose for brachytherapy boost is 20–25 Gy.
- For HDR brachytherapy, four sessions of 10 Gy each are given in 3–4 weeks, with no need for urinary diversion; one or two sessions if brachytherapy is a boost after EBRT, four to five sessions in case of brachytherapy alone.
- By EBRT, the whole pelvis is treated to a dose of 45–50 Gy. A boost of 10–15 Gy is delivered to positive groin nodes through reduced anteroposterior fields.
- One of the limiting factors in the use of external-beam irradiation is the tolerance of the perineal skin.

Volume

Brachytherapy

- The target volume can be defined beginning with tumor volume determination (GTV).
- Many prefer to irradiate the entire length of the urethra, especially in female patients. This is safe for superficial lesions, in which intraluminal irradiation alone is indicated.
- In treating bulky infiltrating lesions with large target volume with interstitial brachytherapy; the risk of sequelae, particularly in penile urethra, is high.

- If brachytherapy is performed after a surgical endourethral resection, the target volume is reduced, allowing brachytherapy for residual disease (postoperative GTV).
- If brachytherapy is indicated as a boost after external therapy, the evaluation of the target volume must take into consideration the initial volume.
- To summarize, the brachytherapy, PTV includes the initial GTV, if given with EBRT, and the postoperative GTV if combined with surgery.
- In all cases, a margin of 1 cm is taken at each extremity of the tumor and a minimal margin of 0.5 cm according to the tumor infiltration (CTV).

Technique of Radiotherapy

Brachytherapy

Intraluminal implant:
- This is performed either with a catheter (closed at the internal part) introduced into the urethra or with a Foley-catheter.
- Both are after-loaded with radioactive sources. With the former, suprapubic urinary diversion is necessary.
- This method is used for very superficial lesions that measure no more than 5 mm in depth.

Interstitial implant:
- This method is more common. The technique of implantation is comparable to that used in the penis and reserved for the penile urethra.
- After introducing a Foley catheter, bevelled hypodermic needles with a length chosen according to the size of the penis are implanted perpendicular to the axis of the organ, equidistant to each other, usually in two planes, one above the urethra and the other one below.
- The different needles are maintained during the time of irradiation by two templates placed laterally to the penis.

- The organ is kept as far as possible from the testis by an adapted sponge.
- In females, both intracavitary and interstitial implants are used; the vagina is used to introduce sources with a vaginal applicator.

External Beam Radiotherapy

In males, radiation therapy for carcinoma of the anterior (distal) urethra is similar to that for penile carcinomas.

Lesions of the bulbo-membranous urethra can be treated with a set of parallel-opposed fields covering the groins and the pelvis, followed by perineal and inguinal boost.

Lesions of the prostatic urethra are treated similar to carcinoma of the prostate.

In females, small meatal or distal urethral lesions are cured with limited therapy. Interstitial implants are usual method for treating meatal carcinomas. Radioactive needles, forming a double-plane or a volume implant, are used. Afterloading implants using ^{192}Ir have replaced radium. For early localized disease without involvement of adjacent organs, a volume implant composed of 8–12 needles arranged in an arc around urethral orifice can be used.

Advanced disease or large tumors extending into the labia, vagina, entire urethra, or base of the bladder cannot be treated with an implant alone and a combination of external-beam irradiation and implant is recommended. The external-beam portal should flash the perineum to cover the entire urethra. The portal should be wide enough to cover the inguinal nodes and should extend superiorly to the L5-S1 interspace to include the pelvic nodes. A bolus may be added to the groins when inguinal nodes are positive.

Sequelae

- Complications due to surgery, irradiation, or combined-modality therapy vary from 0% to 42%.

- Complications include urethral stenosis, fistula, necrosis, cystitis, and hemorrhage. Others may experience incontinence, cystitis, and vaginal stenosis.
- Urethral strictures develop in some patients, necessitating dilatation or urinary diversion.
- Severe complications include fistula formation, bowel obstruction, and, occasionally, operative death.
- In advanced neoplasms, fistula formation may be unavoidable resulting from tumor erosion of adjacent organs and post-radiation tumor necrosis.

PENILE CARCINOMAS

Surgical management is effective in treating penile cancer, but surgery usually means partial or total amputation with subsequent functional disability and psychosexual effect. Radiotherapy has been used to preserve penile function and this approach is the treatment of choice if the rate of local control is comparable to surgery. Penile carcinoma can be cured by radiation but local cure rates and treatment complications vary significantly according to the type of radiotherapy procedure used.

Work-up and Investigations

- *Primary tumor*: Biopsy, urethrocystoscopy.
- *Infiltration can be evaluated by*: Ultrasound and/or CT and/or MRI for the nodes (groin, pelvic and para-aortic areas); whenever possible percutaneous needle aspiration or biopsy of suspicious nodes may be done.
- *Distant dissemination evaluated by*: Chest radiograph, bone scan, liver CT, ultrasonography, as clinically indicated.
- *General laboratory systematic studies*: Blood count and chemistry profile, urinary analysis.

Indication for Radiotherapy

- *Brachytherapy alone:* All tumors, ≤ 4 cm in size, limited to the glans and not extending beyond the balanopreputial sulcus. This differentiation can be difficult if there is accompanying phimosis.
- *Surgery:* Large tumors (>4–5 cm) exceeding beyond glans, partial or total amputation of the penis according to tumor size.
- *External beam radiotherapy:* In cases where there is any contraindication to brachytherapy and/or surgery. Also in case of large tumors where brachytherapy alone is not helpful and patient not accepting any surgical removal of the penis. In these cases, a combination of external beam irradiation plus brachytherapy boost may be administered.
- *In treating lymph nodes by external beam therapy:* First all nodal involvement should be confirmed histologically. Inguinal nodal excision can be performed at the same time as circumcision. One involved node without capsular extension may need no further treatment. If there are several involved nodes with or without capsular extension, adjuvant treatment by external beam irradiation to the groin area ± the iliac nodes is indicated.

Dose of Radiotherapy

- *Radical EBRT or electrons:* 64 Gy in 32 daily fractions given in 6½ weeks.
- *Brachytherapy:* 65 Gy to the 85 percent reference isodose in 6–7 days by LDR. The mean central dose is 75 Gy. The treated volume is dependent on the target volume, mean 50 cucm. For HDR brachytherapy, no data have been published so far. Two schedules may be considered only as proposals: 36 Gy/12 fr/30 days with a boost of 15 Gy/5 fr/11 days one month later, or 54 Gy/27 fr/42 days.
- *Lymph nodes*
  EBRT or electrons: 50 Gy in 25 daily fractions given in 5 weeks.
- *Palliative:* 30 Gy in 10 daily fractions given in 2 weeks.

Volume for Radiotherapy

- CTV encompasses the tumor volume (GTV) plus a margin of 5–20 mm. Since super-infection is very often associated with cancer of the penis, it is sometimes difficult to delineate the exact target volume.
- The target volume must also be defined taking into account the different tumor types.
  - *Superficial tumors:* Thickness, peripheral limits.
  - *Exophytic tumors:* Accurate knowledge of the tumor and its base (depth of implantation).
  - *Infiltrating (± ulcerating) tumors:* Exact topography of the infiltration, depth of the ulceration.
- Very small superficial stage I tumors on the prepuce or glans, unsuitable for surgery or brachytherapy, can be treated with electron therapy as for SCC on the skin. A lead cut-out is made to treat the tumor with a 2 cm margin. An appropriate electron energy and thickness of bolus are chosen to give a skin dose of 100 percent and ensure that the tumor is covered at depth by the 90 percent isodose.
- In larger tumors, CTV is the clinical and radiological GTV with 2 cm margin proximally and distally, that usually gives a PTV covering entire penis.

Technique of Radiotherapy

- The first step of treatment is to perform a wide circumcision, regardless of subsequent surgery or irradiation. This circumcision allows optimal tumor assessment, and consequently better determination of the target volume. It also helps decrease side effects of brachytherapy or external beam radiotherapy.
- The anatomical position of the penile urethra should be marked with a Foley catheter.

External Beam Radiotherapy

- Penis is immobilized by covering with gauze and placed in a central cavity of a wax block within a hinged Perspex box.
- The box is closed, the gauze drawn up through a hole in the top and a wax plug is inserted to maintain the penis in position.
- This wax block allows even build up, and a homogeneous dose is obtained using opposing lateral fields treating iso-centrically with 4 MV or 6 MV photons.
- The testes and groins are shielded by lead shield.
- *For inguinal and pelvic node adjuvant radiotherapy:* Contrast-enhanced planning CT scan is used to define the nodal CTV and a 3D margin of 7–10 mm given for PTV.
- *Conventionally:* Inguinal region field is defined as that extends laterally to the midpoint of the femoral neck, medially to the midline, inferiorly 2 cm below the inferior border of the ischial tuberosity and superiorly to a line joining the top of the anterior superior iliac spine to the pubic symphysis.
- Direct anterior or opposing anterior and posterior beams are used, with central shielding to cover the bladder and MLC shaping. If an anterior electron field is used, an additional margin will be needed to account for the wider penumbra of electrons.
- *In palliative cases:* Radiotherapy can be used to palliate pain and bleeding with a simple beam arrangement to the affected area.

Mould Brachytherapy

- Mould brachytherapy is indicated for very superficial lesions (≤5 mm thick) with well-defined limits. Essentially two types of surface applicators can be used: a personalized one or a standard one.
- The personalized one consists of a mould containing catheters placed according to the tumor topography afterloaded with an iridium source for HDR or LDR brachytherapy. When LDR brachytherapy is applied, the mould must be fixed to the surface of the penis, because of the risk of displacement during irradiation.

- The standard mould is more often used; it is made of two plastic cylinders, the inner one worn over the penis, the outer one containing iridium sources.

Interstitial Brachytherapy

Classical Technique

- The implant is performed under general anesthesia following insertion of a Foley's urinary catheter to localize urethra. Based on the use of hypodermic needles manually after-loaded with iridium wires. The urinary catheter stays in place during the whole irradiation.
- The planning target volume is defined as the GTV (palpable and visible tumor) with a margin of 1–2 cm.
- For small superficial tumors, a single plane implant may be done, but for the majority, the entire circumference of penis is enclosed in two-plane implant. It is usual to use two or three sources in each plane and to maintain parallelism by the use of a small template. The separation between sources is usually 12–15 mm, but it may sometimes be up to 18 mm as determined by the thickness of the shaft of the penis and respecting the rules of the Paris system.
- Hypodermic needles are implanted through the glans, perpendicularly to the axis of the penis.
- During the placement of the needles, two lucite plaques are prepared in the operating room itself. These handmade templates are adapted to each implant. Size, shape and distance of perforations in the template are predetermined according to the position of the needles. The needles are introduced into the corresponding holes of the plaques.

Gerbaulet's Glans Applicator (GAG)

- This system consists of 2 square plates of transparent plastic, 50 mm wide and 2 mm thick. System was designed to ensure parallelism of plates.

- These two identical plates are perforated by holes of 1 mm in diameter, to allow the passage of hypodermic needles; these perforations are located at 5 mm intervals from each other, forming a regular equilateral/triangular-shaped arrangement that is ideal for dose distribution according to Paris system rules.
- At four corners of each plate, there is one hole of 3 mm in diameter, which allows the passage of 4 threaded screws 2.8 mm in diameter and 65 mm in length, made of stainless steel or brass. These threaded screws ensure that the apparatus is held in parallel position, both at the moment of application and during irradiation.
- First plate is positioned alongside lesion on penis and the tumor volume is drawn on the plate. This is then copied on to the other plate. Both plates are then positioned alongside penis with lesion enclosed inside drawn area; and needles implanted through the holes in the plates and through the lesion as per Paris system rules.
- In both these above methods, the shaft of penis is supported erect in a foam block to prevent radioactive material from coming into contact with the skin of the thigh or testes.

Points to Remember

- Systemic antibiotics and circumcision may be needed before radiotherapy to control infection and prevent radiation-induced edema and urethral obstruction.
- Pain and difficulty passing urine are common.
- High fluid intake is encouraged and midstream urine specimens sent regularly to exclude infection.
- Complications of both EBRT and brachytherapy include tissue swelling, moist desquamation, secondary infection, penile ulceration (8%), penile necrosis (3–16%) and urethral strictures (10–45%).

CHAPTER 11

Thyroid Malignancies

Kanika Sharma

ROLE OF RADIOTHERAPY

- Radiation has a modest role and is used infrequently in papillary thyroid cancers.
  - Patients over age 45 with grossly visible extrathyroidal extension at time of surgery.
  - Retrosternal disease locally advanced, otherwise unresectable disease.
  - High likelihood of microscopic residual disease.
  - Patients with gross residual tumor in whom further surgery or radioactive iodine (RAI) would likely be ineffective.
  - Recurrrence after maximum RAI therapy.
- Postoperatively in medullary thyroid cancer and anaplastic thyroid cancers.
- Palliation of metastasis.

ASSESSMENT OF TUMOR

- Symptoms (hoarseness, dysphagia and stridor) and palpation of neck.
- Indirect laryngoscopy to rule out recurrent laryngeal nerve palsy.
- Lateral soft tissue neck X-ray, ultrasonography neck, CT neck.

TARGET DELINEATION

Stage dependent and nodal involvement to be taken into account.

Technique challenging due to contour of the body and possible extension into the mediastinum.

Patient positioning: Supine (with perspex cast from base of skull to mid-thoracic level).

Target Volume

Two to three centimeter margin around the primary tumor and draining lymph nodes.

Spinal cord tolerance to be respected.

Field Placements

Initial AP-PA field with head hyperextended to bring oral cavity out of field.

DTC direct enface field or multifold technique with e^- beam 12–16 MeV.

In medullary thyroid cancer—mini mantle field, chin to T4 lower border.

Field extends from angle of mandible to tracheal bifurcation (entire neck and upper mediastinum). Tissue compensator can be used to account for differences in contour.

Without lymphadenopathy (LAP): Upper border tip of mastoid.

Lower border-sternal notch treated with ant oblique fields.

With lymphadenopathy (LAP): Spinal cord tolerance a concern –20 MeV electron gives ideal distribution or alternately 2 anterior fields centered laterally to spinal cord each rotating through arc of 100–120°.

- Treatment planning with CT and MRI permits evaluation of dose distribution to vital structures.
- Intensity-modulated radiation therapy (IMRT) is also useful in this context.

TUMOR EXTENDING TO SUPERIOR MEDIASTINUM

- Upper margin tip of mastoid
- Lower margin-carina
- Lateral include bilateral deep cervical nodes.

Compensators or wedge in superoinferior dimension improves dose homogeneity.

Dose to the primary site can be escalated after 45–50 Gy by oblique fields.

Mixed beams with posterior photons and anterior electrons or low energy photons can be alternatively used.

Doses: 50 Gy/5 weeks, postmediastinal boost to mediastinal disease 40 Gy/4 weeks.

In postoperative cases dose is 60 Gy in 6–61/2 weeks.

- Gross residual disease requires 68–70 Gy
- Anaplastic thyroid cancer-60 Gy/6 weeks
- Non-Hodgkin's lymphoma of thyroid 35–40 Gy in 4 weeks
- Spinal cord receives 40 Gy/5weeks.

Palliative Radiotherapy

In symptom control of metastatic disease, e.g. vertebral mets 2 vertebrae above and below with direct dorsal spinal field or 2 wedges.

Dose 30–40 Gy in 10–12# in 2–4 weeks.

CHAPTER 12

Irradiation of Blood Products and Spleen

Ashutosh Mukherji

RATIONALE OF IRRADIATION OF BLOOD PRODUCTS

Transfusion associated graft versus host disease is a rare but fatal complication of blood transfusion. It occurs due to leukocyte contamination of whole blood or packed cells (1–2 billion WBCs per unit) or even platelet concentrates (50 million WBCs per unit); for which current methods of filtration are inadequate.

Gamma irradiation inactivates the T-lymphocytes and preserves the function of other blood components.

Indications

Definite Indications

- Allogeneic and autologous bone marrow and peripheral blood stem cell transplant recipients.
- Congenital cellular immunodeficiency disorders.
- Intrauterine and all subsequent transfusions and neonatal exchange transfusions.
- Hodgkin's disease or Non-Hodgkin's lymphoma patients.
- Aplastic anemia patients receiving immunosuppressive therapy.
- Patients receiving purine analogs with associated immuno-suppression.
- Granulocyte transfusions.
- HLA matched single donor platelets.
- Dedicated donations from directed blood relatives.

Possible Indications

- T cell malignancies.
- Patients with B cell malignancies who have received chemotherapy and/or radiotherapy with lymphopenia < 0.5×10^9 cells/L.
- Therapeutic antibodies against T cells.
- Acute leukemias.
- Chronic myeloid leukemia.
- Any patient receiving sufficient high doses of chemotherapy and/or irradiation to cause lymphopenia < 0.5×10^9 cells/L.
- Patients receiving long-term or high dose steroid therapy for malignancies.
- Premature infants weighing less than 1200 g.

Not Indicated in:

- AIDS
- Hemophilia
- Term infants
- Thalassemias
- Congenital humeral immunodeficiency
- Most patients on chemotherapy
- Patients with aplastic anemia not receiving immunosuppressive therapy.

DOSE RECOMMENDATIONS AND TECHNIQUE

- Minimum dose received in the entire irradiated field should be 25 Gy with no part receiving more than 50 Gy.
- Variation allowed for central axis dose is 30% and for periphery is 35%.
- FDA guidelines in USA recommend central axis dose of 25 Gy and minimum of 15 Gy to any other part.
- In UK, recommendation is minimum dose of 25 Gy.
- A double encapsulated gamma source emitter, usually cobalt-60 or caesium-137 is used. The size and shape of outer housing as

well as detail of thickness and material of all housing materials should be properly mentioned. Adequate shielding is done to achieve protection of medical workers.

- Isodose charts are used for dosimetric calculations. These are checked using blood equivalent material in the canister with the canister full. No part of the bag should protrude above the upper rim of canister. Spacers are used to prevent under dosing the canister bottom.
- After calibration, a table is made which shows irradiation times for specified doses.
- In routine use the canisters are filled with blood bags closely packed with any residual spaces filled with small dummy water bags.
- Wipe tests are carried out at frequent intervals (recommended interval is 6 monthly) to detect any leakage of radioactive contamination.

EFFECT OF IRRADIATION ON BLOOD COMPONENTS

Effect on Red Blood Cells

No effect on pH, ATP consumption, 2,3-DPG levels or glucose consumption. There is increased rate of efflux of intracellular potassium.

Effect on Platelets

Function is not significantly affected at doses up to 50 Gy.

Effect on Granulocytes

Available evidence on function derangement is conflicting. But granulocytes should be transfused as soon as possible.

SPLENIC IRRADIATION

Indication for Radiotherapy

- Multiple splenic metastases resistant to chemotherapy.
- Splenomegaly that is painful and caused by chronic lymphocytic, chronic myeloid, hairy cell and prolymphocytic leukemias resistant to standard chemotherapy.
- Painful splenomegaly due to myeloproliferative disorders like polycythemia vera or essential thrombocytopenia.

Dose of Radiotherapy

In case of leukemic infiltration: 0.5–1.0 Gy per fraction per day 2–3 times a week to a total dose of 4–10 Gy, but never more than 20 Gy.

In case of extramedullary hematopoiesis: 0.5–1.0 Gy per fraction several times a week to a total dose of 1–9 Gy.

Volume and Technique of Radiotherapy

- Whole spleen taken as the CTV. Wide margins for PTV not required.
- Attempt to spare left kidney as much as possible.
- As size of spleen decreases, shrinking fields can be used. In cases of extramedullary hematopoiesis; in certain cases, only half the spleen may be treated to prevent severe and protracted myelosuppression.
- Anterior and posterior opposed fields are used.

Points to Remember

- Strict twice to thrice weekly monitoring of blood counts.
- Total dose is decided by level of palliation achieved.
- Cumulative dose to the left kidney is to be monitored.
- Allopurinol to be started to prevent uric acid nephropathy as there can be rapid cell lysis.
- Antiemetic measures should be started.

CHAPTER 13

Palliative Radiotherapy

Vikash Kumar

Aim: *"To cure sometimes, to relieve often and to comfort always".*

BONE METASTASIS

Radiotherapy remains the most effective treatment for relief of metastatic bone pain.

Work-up

- History and physical examination
- HMG, LFT, KFT
- Alkaline phosphatase
- Serum calcium
- Plain radiographs of suspected or symptomatic sites
- Bone scan
- MRI (in cases of cord compression)

Treatment

Local field radiotherapy.

Indications

- Solitary lesions
- Painful lesions
- Weight bearing bones
- Acute spinal cord compression

- Impending pathological fracture
- Pathological fracture after reduction and fixation

Dose: 30 Gy in 10 fractions (It is now realized that single dose of 8 Gy is as good as a fractionated course of 20–30 Gy in 5–10 fractions.

Superficial bones like clavicles, ribs, skull, sacrum may be treated with direct field. The hip joint, shoulder joint and pelvis should be treated with AP-PA portal and dose is prescribed at mid point.

Spine should be treated with patient lying in prone position; depth for dose prescription is 3 cm for cervical spine, 4 cm for dorsal spine and 5 cm for lower dorsal and lumbar spine.

Multiple Symptomatic Metastases

- Radionuclide therapy - Sr-89 or Sm-153
- Hemibody irradiation
  - Upper hemibody irradiation - 6 Gy/1#   ⎤ 4–6 weeks
  - Middle or lower hemibody irradiation   ⎟ apart.
    - 8 Gy/1#   ⎦
- Bisphosphonates
  - Pamidronate 90 mg IV infusion q 4 weekly or
  - Zoledronic acid 4 mg IV q 4 weekly, dose as per creatinine clearance
  - Denosumab 120 mg s/c 4 weelky

BRAIN METASTASIS

Work-up

- History and physical examination
- HMG, LFT, KFT
- MRI Head with contrast/CECT head
- Specific investigations for primary tumor and other metastatic work-up in patients with good PS

Treatment

- Medical decompression: steroids +/– mannitol to be started immediately
- Antiepileptics in patients having convulsions.

Solitary Metastasis

Good PS and Controlled Extraneurologic Disease

- *Resectable:* Surgical excision + postoperative radiotherapy (Usually dose of 45–50 Gy in conventional fraction sizes), SRS
- *Unresectable:* Definitive radiotherapy

Dose of Radiotherapy

- *Definitive:* Depending on histology
- *Palliative:* 30 Gy/10#/2 week

Portal of Radiotherapy

Whole brain radiotherapy using parallel opposed portals.

Patients with KPS < 60, gross neurological deficit, extensive systemic metastasis—symptomatic and palliative care only.

Multiple Metastases

- Patients with KPS ≥ 60:
  Palliative whole brain radiotherapy – 20 Gy/5#/1 week
- Selected cases with good PS and controlled extraneurological disease:
  Surgery + postoperative radiotherapy, or
  Whole brain radiotherapy → boost to tumor

Patients with KPS < 60, gross neurological deficit, extensive systemic metastasis—symptomatic and palliative care only.

LUNG METASTASIS

Indications

Complete occlusion, consolidation or atelectasis, chest wall invasion, brachial plexus involvement, lesions eroding blood vessels leading to hemoptysis and superior vena cava syndrome.

Work-up

- History and physical examination
- HMG, LFT, KFT
- Chest X-ray
- CECT chest (if required for confirmation)

Treatment

Solitary

Good PS and controlled extrapulmonary disease.

- *Resectable:* Surgical resection + disease specific systemic therapy +/– postoperative radiotherapy.
- *Unresectable:* Disease specific systemic therapy.
- Palliative radiotherapy for symptomatic lesions – 20 Gy/5#/1 week by AP-PA portals, calculating the dose at midplane. Field size ranges from 12 cm × 12 cm to 15 cm × 15 cm (with proper lung correction factors).
- *Endobronchial lesions:* HDR brachytherapy 7.5 Gy to 10 Gy 1 cm depth from the mucosa of bronchus.

Multiple

Good PS and controlled extrapulmonary disease:

- Surgery +/– chemotherapy +/– postoperative radiotherapy
- *Unresectable:* Chemotherapy (chemosensitive disease)
- Palliative radiotherapy for symptomatic lesions 20 Gy/5#/1 week

PS < 50, extensive systemic metastasis – palliative care only.

Supportive Treatment

Antibiotics, steroids, bronchodilators and antitussives.

Esophageal Obstruction

Endoluminal due to esophageal growth or extrinsic compression due to lymphoma, germ cell tumor, lung cancer, etc.

Dose: 30 Gy in 10 # by AP-PA portals. Field size is kept minimum to reduce morbidities.

Hemorrhage

Vaginal bleeding due to carcinoma cervix, ca endometrium, hematuria, rectal bleeding, etc.

Dose: 20 Gy in 5 fractions followed by intracavitary hemostatic dose of 30 Gy to surface by LDR brachytherapy.

Orbital Metastasis

Common tumors which metastasize to orbit are breast, lymphomas, leukemias and RCC.

Investigation of choice: Ultrasound B scan, fluorescent angiography.

Dose: 45 Gy in 25 fractions by direct lateral portal at 2.5 cm depth.

Leptomeningeal Metastasis

Useful for areas of CSF flow obstruction or bulky disease.

Dose: 30 Gy in 10 fractions. Craniospinal irradiation is rarely used because of significant toxicity.

CHAPTER 14

Reirradiation

Ashutosh Mukherji

Improvement of radiotherapy (RT) techniques and increase in dose delivered to the tumor in recent times has improved local control; but local disease recurrence after radiotherapy may still occur with or without distant metastasis which can be distressing or even fatal. The choice of an adequate therapy may involve salvage chemotherapy, salvage surgery, or even the repetition of radiation therapy.

Conventional thinking in radiation oncology is that a heavily irradiated tissue will not tolerate re-treatment, but recently this idea has been challenged. Firstly, it is very important to consider the techniques used in the initial treatment (beam energy, volume, doses delivered). Also, the period of time between the two treatments must be taken in consideration as it is postulated that some repair of the initial damage may take place in the interval.

Factors that determine the extent to which residual injury will limit re-treatment tolerance include:

- The amount of cell depletion caused by prior treatment
- The time elapsed since that treatment and therefore the extent of regeneration
- The tissue at risk as high prior doses, short intervals between treatment courses and slow regeneration of target cells will reduce re-treatment tolerance.

Re-irradiation for local recurrence of malignancy after radical radiotherapy has been proven to be of benefit in squamous cell cancers of head and neck but has seldom been used elsewhere.

HEAD AND NECK CANCERS

More than 70% of patients with head and neck cancer present with advanced locoregional disease (stage III and IV). The local or regional failure rates of squamous cell carcinomas of the head and neck range between 20 and 57%. The treatment options include surgery, palliative chemotherapy, supportive care or re-irradiation with or without concurrent chemotherapy. Surgery is the optimal therapy, when disease is amenable to complete resection; however, this is feasible only in a small subset of patients.

Currently, the most common treatment for patients with previously irradiated, unresectable disease is single- or multi-agent chemotherapy with response rates between 10 and 40% and median survivals of 6–8 months. Administration of a second course of radiation to tissues within a previous radiation portal has been previously considered unsafe; but is sometimes feasible in certain cases.

Patients most likely to benefit from re-irradiation are:
- Patients suitable for debulking surgery
- Patients with second primary cancers as opposed to local recurrences
- Primary tumors in the nasopharynx and larynx
- Patients with longer disease free intervals before recurrence.

RESULTS

Brachytherapy

Re-irradiation can also be administered using local interstitial brachytherapy for primary and nodal recurrences.

Radiation Dose and Technique

- Adequate radiotherapy doses are needed for optimal outcomes in radical re-irradiation.

- High doses of re-irradiation are necessary in the radical treatment of recurrent tumor, in view of possibility of radiation resistant clonogens.
- In recurrent nasopharyngeal tumors, 3D-CRT, IMRT, intraluminal brachytherapy and radiosurgery boosts have been used with good results.
- Optimal treatment schedule not yet been defined. Radiation portals must be tight to avoid excessive irradiation of normal tissues. The re-irradiation dose should be optimum, ranging from 60–70 Gy.
- Treatment volumes include CTV = GTV + 1–2 cm. Treatment delivered by multiple beams by conformal RT.

Toxicities

- The most serious is carotid rupture, which occurs in 1–5% of patients, in the setting of re-irradiation. Carotid rupture results in death in almost all instances
- Vascular stenosis and thromboembolism have also been reported
- The incidence of grade 3 and 4 acute mucositis varies between 5 and 32%
- Osteoradionecrosis in 16%
- Cervical fibrosis in 40%
- The frequency of significant hematologic toxicity varies and depends on the chemotherapy regimen used. Regimens such as docetaxel/cisplatin and paclitaxel/cisplatin report grade 3 or worse neutropenia in approximately one third of patients
- Aspects such as quality of life, difficulties with eating, nutrition, speech, pain, fatigue, which are important in weighing the benefit of re-irradiation, still have to be addressed.

USE OF RADIOSURGERY

Recurrent H & N SCC of nasopharynx, maxillary sinus, neck lymph nodes, skull base, nasal cavity, retropharyngeal lymph nodes, orbit can be treated by Cyberknife®. Total doses administered is in the range of 18–40 Gy (median, 30 Gy) in 3 to 5 fractions to the 65–85% isodose line for 3–5 consecutive days. Recent results show fractionated stereotactic radiosurgery is an effective treatment modality as a salvage treatment with good short-term local control.

BREAST CANCER

With large numbers of breast cancer patients being treated with breast conserving surgery followed by systemic therapy and radiotherapy; failure rates after breast conserving therapy (BCT) increase with 1–2% per year and even after mastectomy local recurrence rates might be as high as 40%. The treatment options for locoregional recurrences are limited. Mastectomy or local excision and reconstructive surgery are the preferred therapies; as chemotherapy in presence of radiation induced fibrosis may not be effective. Re-treatment with a second full course of radiation to the whole breast is used with caution as increased toxicity of skin and subcutaneous tissue is feared. In recent years, several investigators reported on re-irradiation either alone or combined with concurrent hyperthermia or chemotherapy.

RADIATION DOSE AND TECHNIQUE

- All patients should undergo computed tomography or FDG18-PET/CT for 3D-CRT planning
- The recommended dose per fraction is 1.8 to 2 Gy in curative intent. Higher doses per fraction can be given in patients expecting a lifetime of only a few months
- The treatment volume comprised all visible lesions or lesions detectable on CT/MRI/FDG-PET/CT or the tumor bed or recurrent tumor.
- With PDR brachytherapy alone, re-treatment doses are biologically a dose of 40 to 50 Gy given within 4 days. It is expected to be more efficient than a conventional fractionated EBRT given within five weeks.

- A novel technique to irradiate patients is intraoperative radiotherapy (IORT) with a 50 kV X-rays source (Intrabeam™) treating patients during surgery and limiting radiation dose to the tumor bed. The dose distribution by the Intrabeam™ source is characterized by a sharp dose fall off, i.e. in 1 cm depth from the applicator surface only 5 Gy is delivered.
- The minimum time interval between first and second radiation treatment should be six months based on published data.
- The minimum second radiation dose in fractionated irradiation should be 40 Gy though higher doses might be possible depending on the treatment volume.
- Re-irradiation can be safely combined with continuous infusion 5-FU or oral capecitabine.
- Possible alternative radiation techniques to fractionated megavoltage external beam therapy are brachytherapy and intraoperative radiation therapy.

Toxicities
- With EBRT, moderate skin and subcutaneous tissue side effects seen with no grade 3 or 4 toxicity. Most commonly noted are erythemas and skin telangiectasias.
- No unacceptable deformities of the breast observed.
- With IORT, mild acute toxicity and no grade 3/4 toxicities.
- Occasional delay in wound healing or wound infection.
- The cosmetic outcome in IORT is good to excellent.
- Hyperthermia may cause skin ulcerations and blisters.

LUNG CANCER
The median time between prior and secondary irradiation around 12 months.

Radiation Dose and Technique
- Prior radiation doses 50 to 70 Gy
- Re-treatment 30 to 60 Gy

- CTV = GTV + 2 cm
- CT/PET based planning

Toxicities

Acute grade 2 and 3 pulmonary toxicity including pleural effusion, radiation pneumonitis, pericardial effusion/pericarditis.

BRAIN TUMORS AND METASTASES TO BRAIN AND SPINAL CORD

Brain and spinal cord, which are late-reacting tissues, have a small α/β value of 2–3 Gy, whereas metastases generally have a larger α/β ratio of 10 Gy. These reference values are reliable for fractionated radiotherapy when the fraction sizes are from 1.2 to 5 Gy. The cumulative biological equivalent dose (BED) should not exceed 140 Gy. In case of spinal cord, early diagnosis of relapse is crucial in conditioning response to re-treatment. An α/β ratio of 1.9–3 Gy could be generally the reference value for fractionated radiotherapy. The cumulative biological equivalent dose (BED) should not exceed 130 Gy. When fraction sizes are up to 5 Gy, the linear-quadratic equation becomes a less valid model. Karnofsky performance status (KPS) >70, age <65 years, controlled primary and no extracranial metastases represent the better prognostic patient class.

Indication for Reirradiation to Brain/Spinal Cord

Reirradiation can be indicated in when the brain/cord metastases cause neurologic symptom/s that can be controlled with re-irradiation.

Reirradiation Questionable for Brain/Spinal Cord

- In-field relapse diagnosed ≤3 months after the first radiotherapy
- Short life expectation of ≤3 months
- Patients with bad performance status (Karnofsky performance status ≤60%)

- Patients with other extra-cranial metastatic sites in progression
- Patients with paresis/plegia and unfavorable histologies (i.e., non small cell lung, kidney, gastrointestinal, head and neck carcinomas, melanoma, sarcomas).

RADIATION DOSE AND TECHNIQUE

- Prior radiation doses 50 to 70 Gy by fractionated RT
- CT/PET based planning
- CTV= GTV + 1–2 cm for brain RT
- If ≥4 metastatic sites, then give WBRT
- If ≤3 metastatic sites, then radiosurgery/FSRT.
- If ≤3 metastatic sites but the tumor diameter is >30 mm, the metastasis is nearby brain stem and/or optical nerves, and/or patient has a long life expectation (i.e. ≥6 months) then FSRT
- Radiation ports for spinal cord should encompass at least two vertebral bodies above and below the level of compression should be designed for treatment.
- With use of Cyberknife in spinal cord metastases, dose of up to 3800 cGy equivalent can be given with risk of myelopathy less than 5%.

Dose Schedule in Brain Metastases

- Re-treatment dose for brain 30 to 40 Gy by fractionated RT.
- *SRS doses:* 24 Gy for tumor volume < 20 mm, 18 Gy for volume 21–30 mm and 15 Gy for volume 31–40 mm.

Dose Schedule in Spinal Cord Metastases

- Ambulant patients and favorable histologies (i.e. breast and prostate carcinomas, lymphomas and seminoma) is 20–24 Gy in10–12 fractions
- Ambulant patients and unfavorable histologies is hypofractionated radiotherapy (e.g. 8 Gy × 2 fractions)
- Patients with paresis/plegia and favorable histologies are hypofractionated radiotherapy (e.g. 8 Gy × 2).

Toxicities

Various toxicities are:
- Focal neurological symptoms (motor and sensory deficits, seizures)
- Complex neuropsychological impairment (learning deficits, intellectual decline, personality changes)
- Cerebrovascular effects (stroke deficits, dementia).
- Leukoencephalopathy
- Telangiectasia and focal hemorrhage in white and gray matter
- Late-onset radionecrosis
- Glial proliferation
- Radiation induced myelopathy risk increases if cumulative dose is > 100 Gy (equivalent dose in 2 Gy fractionation).

BONE METASTASES

Indication for Reirradiation

Patients with painful bone metastases with:
- Long duration from initial treatment (≥4 months)
- Good PS (ECOG: 1–2)
- Solitary bone metastases

Dose Schedule in Bone Metastases

Re-treatment dose ranges from 30 Gy/10 fractions followed by further boost of 10 Gy/5 fractions.

RECTAL CANCERS

Local recurrence of rectal cancer after combined radiation and surgery is fortunately rare. The survival of patients with recurrent or metastatic colorectal cancer usually is less than 12 months and hence re-treatment is essentially palliative in intent; as it is difficult to manage with many of these tumors adhering to or invading into vital pelvic structures.

Radiation Dose and Technique

- Irradiation techniques consist of two lateral fields with/without a posterior pelvic field.
- CTV includes recurrent tumor with a margin of 2–4 cm only.
- Total cumulative doses range from 70 to 100 Gy with a median total dose of 85 Gy.
- Previously irradiated patients with locally advanced colorectal cancer without evidence of distant metastatic disease who are treated with surgical resection before intra-operative electron radiotherapy (IOERT) +/– additional external beam radiotherapy (EBRT). The median IOERT dose is 20 Gy (range from 10–30 Gy).
- But long-term survival is poor due to the high rate of distant metastasis.

TOXICITIES

Late complications include:
- Persistent severe diarrhea
- Small bowel obstruction
- Fistula formation
- Colo-anal stricture
- The main IORT related toxicity is peripheral neuropathy.
- Ureteral narrowing or obstruction.

GYNECOLOGICAL CANCERS

Some 20–40% of patients with advanced primary gynecological tumors are still expected to recur locally. Local control prospects are worse for patients who present with recurrent disease, especially if they have received radiotherapy during the primary management. While 25–50% of selected patients with gynecologic tumors who relapse centrally in an irradiated pelvis can be salvaged by exenteration; post-irradiation recurrences infiltrating the pelvic side wall are not usually considered candidates for exenterative surgery since tumor-free margins cannot be achieved and generally the prognosis of these patients have been fatal.

Radiation Dose and Technique

- Irradiation techniques consist of two lateral fields with/without a posterior pelvic field.
- CTV includes recurrent tumor with a margin of 2–4 cm only.
- Previously irradiated patients with locally advanced cancer without evidence of distant metastatic disease who were treated with surgical resection before intraoperative electron radiotherapy (IOERT) +/− additional external beam radiotherapy (EBRT) The median IOERT dose is 15 Gy (range from 10–20 Gy).
- HDR-brachy to doses of 20–30 Gy.
- The median dose of EBRT that these patients received previously was 53 Gy (range from 40–75 Gy).

Toxicities

Late complications include:
- Persistent severe diarrhea
- Small bowel obstruction
- Digestive tract/urinary fistula formation
- Rectal stricture
- Pelvic infections
- The main IOERT related toxicity is peripheral neuropathy
- Ureteral narrowing or obstruction.

SOFT TISSUE SARCOMAS

For patients with high-grade tumors that fail locally, the outlook is poor with a high probability of metastatic disease; local control remains a major objective, without resort to ablative surgery. Similarly, for patients with recurrent low-grade tumors, further surgical treatment is likely to entail amputation. Re-irradiation offers an alternative approach for both categories of patients.

Radiation Dose and Technique

- Irradiation techniques consist of two opposed fields.
- CTV includes recurrent tumor with a margin of 2–4 cm only.
- IOERT/HDR-brachy to doses of 20–30 Gy.
- EBRT to dose of 20–50 Gy in conventional or hypofractionation.

Toxicities

These include:
- Radionecrosis
- Acute skin reactions and skin ulcerations
- Edema formation, sometimes painful
- Loss of limb function
- The main IORT related toxicity is peripheral neuropathy
- Ureteral narrowing or obstruction for retroperitoneal disease.

CHAPTER 15

Magna Field Radiotherapy

Ashutosh Mukherji

This chapter discusses:
1. Total Body Irradiation
2. Hemibody irradiation
3. Total Scalp Electron Treatment
4. Total Limb Therapy
5. Total Skin Electron Treatment

TOTAL BODY IRRADIATION

Indications

- Total body irradiation (TBI) has been used without stem cell support for palliation of radiation sensitive disease such as chronic lymphocytic leukemia (CLL) or follicular lymphomas.
- Currently, TBI is mainly performed in the context of hematopoietic transplantation for its cytotoxic and immunologic effects. Cytotoxic effect is by contributing to the eradication of any residual cancer; while immunologic effect is by immunosuppression, so that the host does not reject the donor stem cells.

Dose and Technique

- Goal is to deliver as uniform and accurate a dose as possible to the entire body while not exceeding the radiation tolerance of any organs.
- However, dose delivery within ±10% of the prescription dose is standard, while higher dose deviations confined to smaller

volumes particularly in the extremities are acceptable due to large variation in geometry and tissue density throughout the patient's body.

- Use of radiation fields that are larger than the maximum field size (~40 × 40 cm^2) available at standard source-to-surface distance (SSD) treatment distance (~100 cm) in conventional radiotherapy.
- The large photon fields are generally achieved by treating the patient at extended SSD with standard linear accelerators or with special dedicated machines with the conventional collimator removed. On a standard linear accelerator a SSD of 2–5 meter or more is needed to produce a field size large enough to completely encompass most of the patient along the diagonal of a square radiation field.
- Current TBI techniques can be classified into two main groups based on the radiation field size: those that utilize a large field size (**Figs 15.1A to E**) that encompasses the entire patient body and those that use less-than-whole-body field sizes (**Figs 15.2A to C**).
- Patients are irradiated with a parallel-opposed beam configuration. These stationary TBI configurations include single or dual fixed beam dedicated units with patient in supine position and horizontal beams from conventional linear accelerators with patients in supine, upright, or lateral decubitus positions.
- The extended SSD technique using a single large field encompassing the entire patient is by far the simplest and the most prevalent TBI technique used today. These techniques use standard radiotherapy linear accelerators (LINACs) and rely on a maximum collimator setting, a large SSD, and beam divergence to produce the large irradiation field required for TBI. Treatment is typically delivered with a horizontal beam directed towards the primary shielding wall. At SSDs of 500 cm or more, the patient placed along the diagonal of the square field will be completely covered by the radiation.

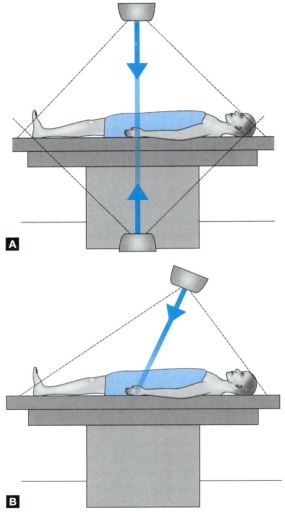

Figs 15.1A and B

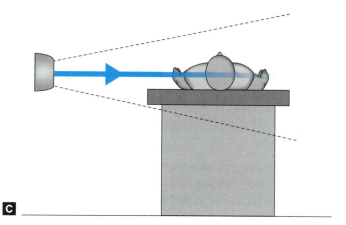

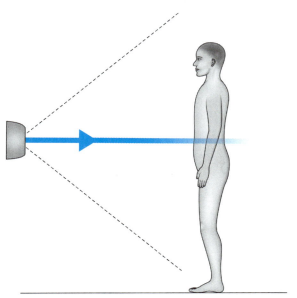

Figs 15.1C and D

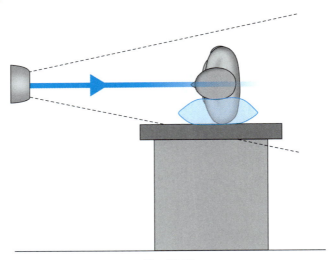

Fig. 15.1E

Figs 15.1A to E Illustration of some of the current large-field total body irradiation techniques in which patient and beams are stationary. (A) Two vertical beams; (B) One vertical beam; (C) One horizontal beam, patient in supine position; (D) One horizontal beam, patient standing or sitting; (E) One horizontal beam; patient in lateral decubitus position

- Doses delivered are 10 Gy in single fraction or 13–16 Gy in 3–5 fractions. Other schedules are 8.5 Gy single dose TBI, 2 Gy × 6 fractions of TBI, and 1.2 Gy × 12 fractions of hyperfractionated TBI.

Dosimetry of TBI

American Association of Physicists in Medicine (AAPM) task group 29 (TG-29) reported on the physical aspects of total and half-body photon irradiation. The general approach recommended by TG-29 in determining the dose delivered to a patient involves three steps:

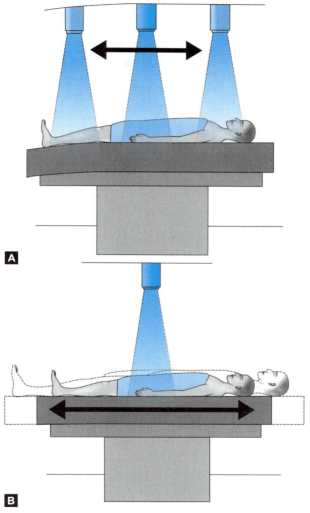

Figs 15.2A and B

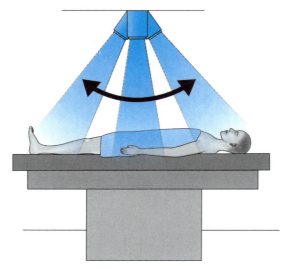

Fig. 15.2C

Figs 15.2A to C Illustrations of some of the small-field total body irradiation techniques in which patient or beam moves. (A) Source scans horizontally; (B) Patient moves horizontally; (C) Sweeping beam

- Absolute dose calibration of the large-field TBI beam at the TBI treatment distance using water or water-equivalent phantoms of a minimum size of 30 by 30 by 30 cm^3
- Dose corrections obtained for a standard phantom that covers entire the beam in full scattering conditions
- Dose corrections for individual size variation in the area of the patient intersecting the beam as well as for patient thickness.

Dose Rates

Dose rate may influence the biologic effects of TBI. Most clinical protocols require low dose rate treatment at the rate of 0.05–0.10 Gy/min.

Patient Positioning

- As treatment times may last up to 30 or 40 minutes for each fraction patients must be in comfortable and reproducible positions.
- AP/PA techniques tend to have more desirable dosimetry and are frequently achievable with horizontal beams.
- With this set-up, patients need to be in lateral decubitus, sitting, or even standing position. An AP/PA technique is best as the dose variation will generally be on the order of ± 7 to 10% owing to a smaller variation in patient thickness in the anteroposterior direction. For adults, lateral fields can have dose variations up to 50% in the head and neck. If compensators are positioned in the head and neck region, care should be taken not to underdose the shoulders by shifting the compensator too far inferiorly.
- Patients receiving TBI are normally not rigidly immobilized, and the compensator material is usually mounted at some distance from the patient.

TBI Boost

- A relative advantage of TBI is the treatment of chemotherapy sanctuary sites. Such regions of the body where there is a higher burden of disease at the time of transplant may be boosted with additional radiation fields to supplement TBI.
- In patients at high-risk for CNS relapse, boost doses of radiation may be delivered to the head, bringing the cumulative cranial dose to 18 Gy (a current standard in children and many adults with ALL). Higher total doses to the head and perhaps the spine can be contemplated in patients being managed for CNS leukemia. Boost doses to the head using lateral fields may be given in 1.8–2.0 Gy fractions.
- Similarly, the testes in males with ALL may be boosted to a cumulative dose of 16–18 Gy. The scrotum may be treated with en face electrons of appropriate energy (or orthovoltage X-rays in young boys).

Toxicities

With Low Dose TBI

Principal side effect is thrombocytopenia, usually occurring after cumulative doses exceeding 1–1.5 Gy. Nausea and vomiting are sometimes observed, controllable by standard antiemetics. When used with alkylating agent chemotherapy, a significant risk (8–9% at 15 years follow-up) of acute leukemia or myelodysplasia has been observed.

With High Dose TBI

Nausea, vomiting, and diarrhea are the most common early side effects when a single fraction of 8–10 Gy TBI is given.

Infectious complications also have a significant role in transplant-related toxicities. Patients also develop dry mouth, a reduction in tear formation, and oral and esophageal mucositis within 10 days.

Reversible alopecia develops at approximately 2 weeks in all patients.

A unique side effect of TBI is parotitis, which usually occurs after the first day of irradiation and subsides within 24–48 hours.

Delayed Toxicity

Lung

Interstitial pneumonitis is the major dose-limiting toxicity for TBI and upper hemibody irradiation (HBI).

Liver

Hepatic venous occlusive disease (VOD) of the liver, an endothelial injury to hepatic sinusoids and hepatocyte injury and hepatic thrombosis are secondary late stage effects. This syndrome, accounting for significant morbidity and mortality is characterized by hepatic enlargement, ascites, jaundice, encephalopathy, and weight gain in 10–40% of patients.

Lens

There is a high intrinsic radiation sensitivity of the lens. Lens shielding during TBI is not recommended because of the risk of retro-ocular relapse of leukemia, but is a consideration in aplastic anemia and other non-neoplastic disease managed with stem cell transplantation.

Kidney

Doses over 12 Gy are associated with increased risks of nephropathy.

Growth, Gonadal and Endocrine Effects

Almost all children who undergo bone marrow transplantation with TBI experience decreased growth velocity, which is less with fractionated than single dose TBI. High-dose TBI produces primary gonadal failure in almost all patients, but recovery may occur. In children, puberty is usually delayed. Thyroid dysfunction is reported in as many as 43% of patients after TBI.

Secondary Cancers

The risk for development of a second tumor 10–15 years after intensive chemoirradiation and stem cell transplantation is estimated to be approximately 20%. Myelodysplastic syndrome and acute myeloid leukemia (AML) are the most common secondary tumors in patients treated for lymphoid malignancies. Patients who are older, who experienced acute graft versus host disease (GVHD) treated with antithymocyte globulin or anti-CD3 antibodies, or who receive TBI are at greatest risk.

HEMIBODY IRRADIATION

Indications

- Palliate widely metastatic solid tumors.
- Patients with multiple painful osseous metastases. The pain relief produced by single fraction Hemibody irradiation (HBI) for skeletal metastases involving several sites is fast, with nearly 50% of all patients responding within 48 hours and 80% within 1 week after treatment. The duration of pain relief persists for at least 50% of the patient's remaining life.
- Planned sequential upper and lower HBI 6–8 weeks apart has been used to treat multiple myeloma, malignant lymphoma, and other widely disseminated tumors.
- HBI appears to be capable of delaying the progression of existing asymptomatic metastasis and the clinical development of new metastases.

Dose and Technique

- The most effective HBI doses found by the Radiation Therapy Oncology Group (RTOG) study are 6 Gy for upper HBI and 8 Gy for lower and middle HBI. When treatment of the other half of the body is indicated, it is advisable to wait 6–8 weeks to allow a sufficient recovery of blood cells and irradiated marrow to take place.
- HBI can often be delivered on a conventional linear accelerator using extended distances. Subtotal body irradiation is usually divided into upper HBI, lower HBI, and middle HBI.
- An arbitrary line at the bottom of L4 vertebral body is commonly used to separate upper and lower HBI.
- Treatment is delivered using AP/PA parallel-opposed fields. The patient is positioned with a vertical beam allowing coverage of the hemibody, and the treatment table is lowered to the appropriate level or to the floor.

- Shielding of previously irradiated areas or other body regions to reduce toxicity, such as the salivary glands and the lungs, may be employed.
- The dose is prescribed to the midplane of the patient at the central axis of the beam.

Complications

- The most common side effects associated with single-dose HBI are nausea and vomiting, mainly when the abdomen is included within the fields. Premedication with steroids and antiemetics is required.
- Since most of the patients are frequently anorectic or cachectic from their underlying illness, dehydration and need for intravenous fluids is common with HBI.
- Diarrhea occurs commonly when a significant volume of the intestines is irradiated and may last for several days. The severity of this side effect can be reduced by limiting the dose to the abdomen to 6 Gy.
- The risk of pneumonitis is very low if the single fraction uncorrected dose to the whole lungs is limited to 7 Gy. If 8 Gy is delivered to the upper body, partial transmission lung blocks to limit the lung dose at 6–7 Gy is recommended.

TOTAL SCALP IRRADIATION

Indications

- Total scalp irradiation is sometimes necessary in the management of malignancies (e.g. cutaneous lymphoma, melanoma, and angiosarcoma) that present with widespread involvement of the scalp and forehead.
- Goal is to deliver a uniform dose to the scalp with minimal dose to underlying brain.

Dose and Technique

- A simple technique that abuts lateral electron fields to parallel opposed photon fields, the latter of which treats the rind of the scalp while avoiding brain tissue is used.
- The outer edge of the electron field overlaps the inner edge of the 6 MV X-ray field by 3 mm to account for the divergence of the contralateral 6 MV X-ray field.
- As the electron and X-ray penumbras are not matched, their common border is moved 1 cm toward beam center halfway through treatment to improve dose homogeneity.
- Initially, the common border is set at approximately 0.5 cm inside the inner table of the skull. Moving the common border further toward the inner table of the skull reduces brain irradiation at the expense of the X-ray beam being replaced by an electron beam that would begin to graze the skull and grazing radiation penetrates less deeply, possibly underdosing the scalp in this region.
- This technique is straightforward to plan and implement but hot spots along the midline superior brain tissue plane is a concern. Dose delivered is between 20 and 30 Gy.

TOTAL LIMB IRRADIATION

Indications

- Irradiate the superficial anatomy of a limb for management of cancer (e.g. melanoma, lymphoma, Kaposi's sarcoma).
- If the depth beneath the surface is 2 cm or less, electrons offer a uniform dose while sparing deep tissues and structures.

Dose and Technique

- Six equally spaced 5-MeV electron beams are used to irradiate a 9 cm diameter cylinder. Each beam is sufficiently wide, so that the entire circle falls within the uniform portion of each beam.

- Tangential radiation to the surface of the cylinder delivers a greater dose as a result of oblique incidence and at the same time, tangential radiation penetrates less deeply.
- The utilization of six or more beams begins to simulate 360° arc therapy. This results in the average maximum dose along each radius being approximately 2.5 times the given dose of each of the six fields.
- By this method, 90% of the average maximum dose penetrates 8–10 mm, less than the value of 15 mm for a single beam incident normally on a flat surface. Also, the surface dose increases to 90% or more of average maximum dose compared with approximately 70% of the given dose for a single beam incident normally on a flat surface (*Self-bolusing effect of tangential electron radiotherapy*).

TOTAL SKIN IRRADIATION

Indications

- Total skin electron irradiation is a modality designed for management of diseases that require irradiation of the entire skin surface or a significant portion of it.
- It is used most frequently for treatment of mycosis fungoides.

Dose and Technique

- Technique used is the modified Stanford technique. Implementation of this technique is estimated at 105 hours. The radiation therapy accelerator should have a high dose rate mode and interlocks for electron energy, gantry angle, and X-ray jaws.
- It also requires an external patient stand with a plastic diffuser, an external scattering foil to broaden the beam, special dosimetry equipment for quality assurance and calibration and special shields for selected parts of the patient.

- First, the treatment requires a broad beam from right to left, which can be achieved by a combination of treating the patient at an extended SSD (300–400 cm). The beam is made uniform from head to foot by abutting two fields at the 50% off-axis ratio. The 50% off-axis ratio lies outside the edge of the light field, so when properly abutted, there is a gap between the edges of the respective light fields.
- By aiming the beams up and down, the largest Bremsstrahlung contribution (central axis) misses the patient. The dose is made uniform around the circumference of the patient by irradiating from six different directions and this tangential radiation results in a higher surface dose and a less penetrating dose.
- Placed upstream of the patient is a plastic screen that serves as both an energy degrader and a scatterer.
- Dose homogeneity is also dependent on patient position, and reproducing the positions of the Stanford technique is important.

Boost and Shielded Areas

- Since there always will be areas that are underdosed (e.g. top of scalp, sole of feet, perineum, and under the breast or under the panniculus of obese individuals); these areas and sometimes tumorous lesions require separate treatment and boosting, respectively.
- In contrast, fingers, feet, and toes typically receive excess dose and are shielded for a portion of the treatment.

CHAPTER 16

Bone and Soft Tissue Tumors

Kanika Sharma

BONE TUMORS

Role of Radiation Therapy

Although surgery is the treatment of choice, radiotherapy may be used to control primary disease.

It is treatment of choice in sites where surgery is not possible due to inaccessibility or where amputation would be necessary for local control.

It may be used in patients with metastatic disease where palliation of symptoms is required.

Assessment of Primary Tumor

X-ray of bone lesions is required to localize tumor and assess bone stability.

CT and MRI define extent of disease and also delineate associated soft tissue masses.

Isotope bone scans can exclude lesions in other bones.

Metastatic lung disease should be ruled out.

Target Delineation

Target Volume

- *Osteosarcoma:* Tumor volume identified by imaging with a margin of 2–3 cm around that tumor.

- *Ewing's sarcoma:* Generous margin of 3–5 cm around the original tumor volume.
- *Giant cell tumor and histiocytosis:* 1 cm margin around the primary tumor.

  Immobilization should be assured by using perspex cast, vacuum bag, alpha cradle, foot rest and arm pole.

  Ensure that where possible the scar is placed at right angles to the incident beam.

Radiotherapy Technique

Field Placements

- For limb lesions, opposing fields are normally used.
- The fields should not cross adjacent joints unless it is necessary to do so in order to cover the tumor.
- Field edges should be preferably at well-defined bony margins.
- In the pelvis, care should be taken to exclude bladder and bowel as much as possible.
- Spinal cord doses should be minimized by using electron field, shallow wedged fields or rotational techniques as possible.

Beam energy: Cobalt
         6 MV X-rays

Dose Prescription

- *Osteosarcoma:* 54–66 Gy in 27–33 fractions over 5.5–6.5 weeks at a dose rate of 2 Gy per fraction treated five days a week.
- *Ewing's sarcoma:* 55 Gy in 27 fractions given in 5.5 weeks at a dose rate of 2 Gy per fraction treated five days a week.
- *Giant cell tumor:* 45 Gy in 23 fractions given in 4.5 weeks at a dose rate of treated five days a week.
- *Palliative treatment (uncontrolled metastatic disease):* Hypo-fractionated radiotherapy as per the need.

SOFT TISSUE SARCOMAS

Role of Radiation Therapy

In downstaging inoperable tumors where complete excision is otherwise not feasible.

Sites where surgery is not possible due to inaccessibility.

Where metastasis is present and surgical excision of primary will result in unacceptable functional or cosmetic defect.

Postoperative, where there are:

- Close or positive resection margins, i.e. incomplete or marginal resection.
- High-grade tumor.
- Positive regional lymph nodes.

Assessment of Primary Tumor

- Clinical examination.
- MRI helps to identify the extent of tumor and edema in muscles.
- Surgical findings.

Target Delineation

Target Volume

- Defined by pretreatment MRI scans.
- Alternatively, CT scans may be used where MRI unavailable.
- Biopsy incisions and needle tracks should be included within the treatment volume.
- Immobilization should be assured by using perspex cast, vacuum bag, alpha cradle, foot rest and arm pole.
- Ensure that where possible, the scar is placed at right angles to the incident beam.

Radiotherapy Technique

Field Placements

Grossly identified tumor with 5 cm margin in grade I tumors.

With 8 cm margin in grade II and III tumors.

A margin of 2–3 cm is sufficient during boost therapy.

It is preferable to spare an uninvolved compartment from full dose treatment in order to preserve lymphatic drainage.

Shrinking fields may be used to deliver high dose to the primary.

For limb lesions, opposing fields are normally used.

The fields should not cross adjacent joints unless it is necessary to do so in order to cover the tumor.

In the pelvis, care should be taken to exclude bladder and bowel as much as possible.

Spinal cord doses should be minimized by using electron field, shallow wedged fields or rotational techniques as possible.

In high-grade lesions local control advantage may be obtained by using postoperative brachytherapy.

Beam energy: Cobalt

6–10 MV X-rays

Dose Prescription

Preoperative Radiotherapy

The 50 Gy/5 weeks/25 fractions

Followed by surgery

Boosted with brachytherapy 16–20 Gy

or IORT 12–16 Gy

or EBRT

14 Gy in negative margins

16–18 Gy with microscopic positive margins

20–26 Gy in gross residual disease

Langerhan's cell histiocytosis—8–10 Gy in 4–5 fractions given in one week.

Postoperative Radiotherapy

The 54–66 Gy in 27–33 fractions given in 5.5–6.5 weeks at a dose rate of 2 Gy per fraction treated five days a week.

Palliative Treatment (Uncontrolled Metastatic Disease)

The 40–50 Gy in 15 fractions given in 3 weeks at dose rate of 2.5–3.5 Gy per fraction treated five days a week.

CHAPTER 17

Radiotherapy of Nonmalignant Diseases

Ashutosh Mukherji

PRINCIPLES FOR USING RADIOTHERAPY IN NONMALIGNANT DISEASES

- To estimate natural course of disease.
- Potential consequences of nontreatment.
- Review alternate therapies and their results.
- Risk-benefit analysis.
- Proof of failure of other conventional therapies and that indication is justified.
- Individual potential long-term radiogenic risks.
- Inform patient of all details of radiotherapy; to take informed written consent; assurance of long-term after care as well as provision of competent second opinion.

  Various sites where radiotherapy is used in treating non-malignant diseases are: Central nervous system (CNS), head and neck, eye and orbit, skin and connective tissue, skeletal system.

Meningiomas

These make up 15–20% of all primary brain tumors. Treatment of choice is radical surgical resection.

Indications for Radiotherapy

- Residual tumor after subtotal resection.
- Tumor relapses after previous surgery.

- Inoperability due to proximity to critical brain structures.
- Co-morbid conditions precluding surgery.

Recommendations and Dose of Radiotherapy

- Primary radiotherapy in surgically inoperable cases.
- Radiation therapy (RT) postoperatively after incomplete resection.
- In case of WHO, grade II/III tumors.

Benign Meningiomas

Treatment volume is GTV + 1 cm margin.

Total dose given is 54 Gy in 1.8–2.0 Gy per fractions over 5.5–6 weeks.

Malignant Aggressive Meningioma

Treatment volume is GTV + 2–3 cm margin.

Total dose given is 60 Gy in 1.8–2.0 Gy per fractions over 6.5–7.5 weeks.

SRS/SRT/IMRT can be used to treat smaller lesions or those lying near critical organs.

Pituitary Adenomas

Therapeutic options include surgery, radiotherapy, drugs or surveillance.

Indications for Radiotherapy

Always given postoperatively:

- After subtotal resection.
- Tumor relapses after previous surgery.
- In clinically relevant persisting hormone secretion even after surgery.

*Recommendations, Volume, Technique
and Dose of Radiotherapy*

- Primary RT in surgically inoperable cases. Total dose given is 45–50 Gy in 1.8 Gy per fraction for 6 weeks.
- Adjuvant RT, postoperatively after incomplete resection.
- MRI- or CT-based planning is done.
- 6–18 MV photons are used.
- *In fractionated RT:* Total doses are 45 Gy (microadenomas) and 50.4 Gy (macroadenomas) @ 1.8 Gy per fraction. Dose to rest of chiasma and pituitary gland is kept below 50 Gy, to brain tissue below 60 Gy and to brainstem below 50 Gy.
- *In radiosurgery:* Total doses are >12–13 Gy (for nonsecreting and inactive adenomas) and 15 Gy (for all other adenomas). Dose to rest of chiasma and pituitary gland is kept below 8 Gy and to 10 mL of brain tissue below 10 Gy.

Craniopharyngiomas

It has been covered in pediatric CNS chapter.

Acoustic Neuromas

It is covered in CNS chapter.

Arteriovenous Malformations

It has been covered in CNS chapter.

Chordomas

These are rare slow growing midline tumors, originating from embryonal notochord rest in base of skull, clivus, vertebral column or sacral region. Complete surgical excision is the treatment of choice.

Indications for Radiotherapy

- Inoperability
- After incomplete resection.

Dose: More than 65 Gy.

Proton beams, gamma knife or intensity-modulated radiation therapy (IMRT) are particularly useful in treating small tumors near vital structures.

Juvenile Nasopharyngeal Angiofibroma

This is a rare, benign vascularized tumor in the head and neck, mainly affecting males; and develops in the sphenoethmoidal suture and spread from epipharynx and nasal cavity to the sphenopalatine foramen and pterygopalatine fossa. Intracranial spread occurs in 25% of cases. Surgery combined with embolization is the treatment of choice.

Indications for Radiotherapy

- Stage IV tumor with intracranial spread.
- Residual tumor after subtotal resection.
- Tumor relapses after previous surgery.
- Tumor rests.

Recommendations, Volume, Technique and Dose of Radiotherapy

- Primary RT in stage IV cases. Total dose given is 55 Gy in 1.8 Gy per fraction for 6 weeks.
- MRI- or CT-based planning is done.
- 6–18 MV photons are used.
- Fractionated stereotactic radiotherapy (SRT) or IMRT used to protect vital structures.

Pterygium

It is a wing-shaped fibrovascular proliferating tissue at the border between conjunctiva and cornea originating mostly from the medial corner of the eye. Corneal involvement can lead to blindness. Complete surgical excision is the treatment of choice.

RT indicated in: Preoperative, primary treatment, relapse after surgery.

Doses: 10 Gy per week × 6 such fractions/25 Gy single fraction using orthovoltage machines or strontium-90 brachytherapy.

Choroidal Hemangioma

These are slow growing benign tumors originating from the choroidal vessels. Photodynamic therapy with verteporfin is the treatment of choice especially in lesions away from the center.

Radiotherapy Indicated in

- Nonresponding cases
- Lesions in proximity to macula or papilla.
- In advanced cases, to maintain the eye as a whole.

Recommendations, Volume, Technique and Dose of Radiotherapy

- Earlier the RT starts, the better.
- In localized type (age 30–50 years), total dose recommended is 18–20 Gy in 10 fractions of 1.8–2.0 Gy each.
- In diffuse type (age 5–10 years), total dose recommended is 30 Gy in 15 fractions.
- Head mask and vacuum contact lenses used for better eye fixation.
- Brachytherapy used in localized lesions. Iodine-125, cobalt-60 and ruthenium-106 are used; of which Iodine-125 is preferred. Dose delivered is 30–240 Gy from apex to base of lesion.

Age-related Macular Degeneration

This is one of the leading causes of blindness in developed countries. Nicotine abuse is an important risk factor. Typical signs are: (a) drusen (yellow spots of cellular detritus), (b) retinal pigment epithelium changes, (c) serous or hemorrhagic retinal detachment, and (d) choroidal neovascularization.

Recommendations, Volume, Technique and Dose of Radiotherapy

- Protons and brachytherapy with ruthenium-106, palladium- 103 and strontium-90 are used; these provide protection for eye structures.
  Dose: Photons 2 Gy fraction to a total dose of 12–16 Gy (maximum 20 Gy) or 4–5 fractions of 4 Gy each to a total dose of 20 Gy
  Protons: 2 fractions to a total dose of 20–24 CGE.
- Photon therapy using linear accelerator with mask fixation via lateral semicircular field is also used. The unaffected eye is spared by 10-degree posterior gantry tilt.

Endocrine Orbitopathy (Graves' Disease)

It is an autoimmune inflammatory fibrosing eye disease related to hyperthyroidism, toxic struma and Hashimoto's thyroiditis. Auto antibodies are formed against TSH receptors in eye muscles; leading to their inflammation and fibrosis, causing edema and proptosis.

Radiotherapy Indicated in

- Medium dose RT in progressive and recurring disease.
- Low dose RT is very effective in early inflammatory disease.

The goals of RT are:
- Bring about clinical remission.
- Reduce/eliminate functional deficits.
- Improve cosmesis.
- Avoid or decrease side effects of other treatment modalities like surgery, long-term steroids, immunosuppressives like cyclosporine, plasmapharesis.

Volume, Technique and Dose of Radiotherapy

- Both orbits are irradiated by opposing lateral opposing fields with 6–10 MV photons to a dose of 20 Gy in 10 fractions.
- CT planning done.
- Half beam block or lateral fields with 10-degree posterior tilt used to spare opposite lens/posterior eye chamber.
- Blocks are used to spare paranasal sinuses and intracranial structures.
- The central beam and anterior field border is daily adjusted to 5–6 mm behind iris or pupil on both sides.
- The posterior field border covers the ring of Zinn at superior orbital fissure.

Diseases of Tendons and Joints

RT is a last resort approach after failure of all other noninvasive treatments, but before surgery. There is reduction of pain, but the pathomorphologic changes are not removed.

Recommended doses are: 0.5–3.0 Gy daily doses for acute inflammation, 2–3 times a week; and up to 6 Gy for chronic inflammation. If response is seen, a second course is repeated after 6 weeks.

Indications for RT

Degenerative osteoarthritis: Affected joints are irradiated by enface or opposing fields using orthovoltage (150–200 kV) or low energy photons (6 MV). Dose reference point is at the center of the joint.

Tendonitis and Bursitis

- *Rotator cuff syndrome:* Using orthovoltage machine (200–250 kV). Opposing fields are used. Dose reference point is at the center of the joint.

- *Tennis/Golfer's elbow:* Using orthovoltage machine (200–250 kV) or low energy photons, opposing fields are used. Dose reference point is at a depth of 5 mm.

Calcaneodynia/achillodynia: Pain syndromes of heel and Achilles' tendon. Affected area is treated by orthovoltage (100–150 kV) or low energy photons, using stationary (plantar area) or opposing (dorsal area) fields to deliver a dose of 0.5–1.0 Gy × 3–6 fractions. Dose reference point is at depth of 5 mm for plantar field and at center of joint for dorsal field.

Desmoid (Aggressive Fibromatosis)

These are benign connective tissue disorders of deep muscular aponeurotic structures in muscle fascias, aponeuroses, tendons and scar tissues. These are of two types: extra- and intra-abdominal. Surgical removal with a margin of 2–5 cm is treatment of choice.

Radiotherapy is indicated in

- Inoperable cases
- After R2 resection.
- After R1 resection if repeat surgery is done.
  Total dose recommended for primary RT is 65 Gy @ 2 Gy per fraction; while postoperatively recommended dose is 55 Gy @ 2 Gy per fraction.

Keloids and Hypertrophic Scars

These are excessive tissue proliferation around scars after skin injury caused by surgery, burns, chemicals, and inflammation or even spontaneous.
  Recommended total dose is 40 Gy @ 2 Gy per fraction.

Heterotropic Ossification

- It consists of real bone located in the periarticular soft tissue; and about one third of all patients with this condition have undergone total hip replacement. It is thought to originate from pluripotent mesenchymal stem cells in periarticular tissue developing into osteoblastic stem cells.

- Prophylactic RT (in postoperative period, 24–48 hours after surgery). Dose recommended is 6–7 Gy in single fraction.
- Preoperative RT of 7 Gy in single fraction is recommended.
- Target volume includes the typical localizations of heterotropic ossification with cranial border 3 cm above acetabulum and lower border including two-third of shaft. The dose reference point is central beam at the center of the target volume (at about 8–12 cm depth).

Morbus Peyronie

- This is a chronic, usually progressive, inflammatory tissue proliferation of the penile tunica albuginea; affecting men between 40 and 60 years age.
- At first, inflammatory changes occur, followed by connective tissue reaction and formation of hard plaques, lumps or cords; which can spread to involve entire penile shaft.
- RT is best given in early stages and delays induration; leading to reduction in pain, bends and function loss.
- It is given with gonad separation; with sparing of glans penis.
- Flaccid penis is treated via dorsal field with orthovoltage machine or using 6 MeV electrons with 5–10 mm bolus.
- HDR brachytherapy used in cases with extensive induration.
- Total dose recommended is 20 Gy in 10 fractions @ 2 Gy per fraction. Hypofractionated RT can also be given with dose 12–15 Gy in 3–4 fractions.

Morbus Dupuytrens and Morbus Ledderhose

- Connective tissue disorders affecting palmar and plantar aponeurosis.
- Prophylactic use in early stages shows good response.

- Target cells are proliferating fibroblasts and inflammatory cells.
- *Goal:* Avoid further progression and later surgery.
- 100–150 kV orthovoltage and 6 MeV electrons used in treating.
- Margin of 1 cm laterally, 2 cm proximally and distally is given to avoid field edge recurrences.
- Dose recommended is 20–30 Gy in 10–15 fractions @ 2 Gy per fraction.
- End point of therapy is softening of lumps and strands with improvement in function.

CHAPTER 18

Emergency Radiotherapy

Kanika Sharma

SUPERIOR VENA CAVA OBSTRUCTION (SVCO)

- First reported by William Hunter in 1757.
- Caval obstruction may be an incidental finding on CT scan or may be the fulminant, initial presentation of a malignancy.
- Malignant causes account for more than 90% of cases.
- Bronchogenic carcinomas, both small cell (SCLC) and non-small cell (NSCLC) are responsible for 65–80% of cases; while mediastinal tumors, particularly thymoma and thyroid cancer, account for 20% of malignant cases.

Treatment

- Includes mainly radiotherapy and chemotherapy, as well as endovascular stenting and medical decompression. Overall prognosis is poor, especially for those with lung cancer.
- Chemotherapy is indicated in chemo-sensitive tumors such as small cell lung cancer, lymphoma, leukemia and germ cell tumors.
- Radiotherapy is indicated in non-small cell lung cancer and other less chemo-sensitive tumors and when SVC stenting is not available.
- The GTV is defined on the CECT scans to include tumor mass and the site of SVCO. The CTV is chosen according to tumor type and patterns of spread. The CTV to PTV margin is 1–2 cm.

Doses Prescribed

- 20 Gy in 5 daily fractions of 4 Gy given in 1 week or 30 Gy in 10 daily fractions of 3 Gy given in 2 weeks by direct or AP-PA fields.
- For some chemo-sensitive tumors, a single fraction of 4 Gy in conjunction with chemotherapy may give adequate immediate palliation.
- Patients with lung cancer have an overall 5-year survival of only 2%, compared with a 10% survival for those with breast cancer and a 40% survival for patients with lymphoma. Median survival is typically only 6 to 9 months following treatment.

MALIGNANT SPINAL CORD COMPRESSION

Malignant spinal cord compression (MSCC) is presently the only defined indication for emergency radiotherapy. Spinal cord compression from epidural metastases occurs in 5–10% of cancer patients, and in up to 40% of patients with pre-existing nonspinal bone metastases.

Clinical Features

- Symptoms depend on location of the compression.
- Anterior tumors can cause compression by growing posteriorly from the vertebral body into the epidural space, or by vertebral body collapse. Lateral and posterior elements are less common.
- Paravertebral tumors can cause compression by entering the spinal canal through the intervertebral foramina.
- Lesions at the conus medullaris can produce symptoms like saddle anesthesia, acute urinary retention, incontinence of bowel and bladder, and impotence. Motor weakness and spasticity are also seen.
- A tumor involving the lateral corticospinal tracts can cause weakness, spasticity, hyper-reflexia, and an extensor plantar response (Babinski's sign).

- A lesion involving the lateral spino-thalamic tract causes numbness, paresthesias, and decreased temperature sensation over the contralateral limb or trunk below the lesion; producing the classic finding of absence of perspiration or of temperature (cold) sensation.
- A lesion in the posterior column can cause gait ataxia seen by Romberg's sign. Paresthesias can occur below the level of the lesion.
- Cauda equina lesions cause radicular pain in the thigh, weakness, and atrophy of muscles. Saddle anesthesia, absent ankle reflexes, impotence, urinary urgency, or acute retention and constipation are also seen.
- Bladder symptoms include hesitancy, dribbling, incontinence, urgency with incontinence, or acute retention. Loss of bladder control is seen early in the presentation of tumors in or below the conus and later in tumors above the conus.
- Cord lesions above L1 can lead to impotence or reflex priapism. Lesions involving S2–S4 may produce loss of erection and ejaculation ability. Decreased genital sensation can occur from lesions affecting the S2 nerve roots.

Treatment

- The most important modality for imaging of suspected MSCC is contrast MRI.
- Management can be Medical, Surgical or by Radiotherapy. With treatment, the median overall survival ranges from 3–16 months.
- Medical decompression means treating with dexamethasone given at an initial dosage of 16 mg divided into four daily doses, with subsequent taper over next few weeks.
- Surgical decompression is by either laminectomy with or without kyphoplasty for posterior situated tumors or vertebral body resection for anterior tumors.

- The indications for surgery are:
  - unknown primary tumor
  - unstable spine or vertebral displacement
  - relapse following spinal radiotherapy
  - neurological symptoms which progress during radiotherapy
  - relatively radio-resistant tumor
  - paralysis of rapid onset.
- Palliative radiotherapy most commonly to a dose of 30 Gy in 10 fractions is useful in cases not amenable to surgery after starting medical treatment. Shorter therapy courses are also used and provide similar pain relief but have decreased long-term recurrence free rates.

Technique and Target Volume for Radiotherapy

- The patient is planned and treated ideally in the prone position using a direct posterior beam.
- The GTV includes vertebral and soft tissue tumor as seen on CT planning scan and diagnostic MRI.
- The CTV includes the spinal canal, the width of the vertebra and one vertebra above and below the SCC if the planning is based on MRI, or two vertebrae above and below if based on X-ray or CT.
- The CTV to PTV margin is 1 cm. To treat the PTV adequately at depth, a direct 6 MV photon beam may be used. For lumbosacral lesions, a better dose distribution may be obtained with opposing beams.
- The field edge defined at the simulator to cover the PTV represents the 50 per cent isodose.
- The dose prescription point is the depth of the anterior spinal canal. This is usually at 5–7 cm in the cervical and thoracic region, and at 7–8 cm in the lumbar region.

Doses Prescribed

Palliative

- 20 Gy in 5 daily fractions of 4 Gy given in 1 week.
- 30 Gy in 10 daily fractions of 3 Gy given in 2 weeks.
- A single dose of 8 Gy may be used for palliation of pain in patients with established paraplegia for more than 24 h.

Radical

- *Solitary plasmacytoma:* 45 Gy in 25 daily fractions of 1.8 Gy given in 5 weeks.
- *Lymphoma:* 30–36 Gy in 15–18 daily fractions given in 3–3½ weeks.

BONE METASTASES

- The most common tumors to metastasize to bone are prostate, breast and lung cancers.
- Emergency treatment is started in conditions of acute bone pain, impending or pathological fractures, and spinal cord compression by adjacent bone disease and may involve surgery and or radiotherapy.
- Surgical management is primarily to prevent or treat pathologic fractures. The goals are to prevent or relieve pain, improve motor function, and to improve overall quality of life. Treatment is more effective when the procedure is performed prophylactically. Various procedures include vertebroplasty, laminectomy, arthroplasty and hemiarthroplasty, internal fixation by plating or nailing.
- The use of bisphosphonates has shown to both decrease local pain and cause apoptosis of cancer cells.
- Radiation therapy also has been reported to be effective in palliating painful bone metastases, with partial pain relief seen in 80–90% of patients, and complete pain relief in 50% of patients.

- Multiple dose regimes like 30 Gy in 10 fractions, 15 Gy in 5 fractions, 20 Gy in 5 fractions, 25 Gy in 5 fractions and 8 Gy single fraction have been used.
- For patients with a poor performance status, extensive non-osseous metastases, and/or a short life expectancy, the most appropriate treatment is a single fraction of 8 Gy.
- For patients with a longer life expectancy, bone-only metastases, and good performance status; a longer course of treatment (30 Gy in 10 fractions) may be required.

Target Volume and Technique of Radiotherapy

- Where possible, the whole structure should be treated. It is usual to include one or two vertebrae above and below the site of involvement.
- When treating a bone postoperatively, the entire prosthesis or intramedullary nail should be covered with a margin of normal bone. This is the area most at risk of residual tumor.
- In patients with multiple painful bone metastases, wide field half-body volumes can be treated.
- When planning the treatment volume, a margin must be added to ensure the target volume is covered by the 90–95 per cent isodose.
- Anterior and posterior opposing beams are used for larger fields.
- The prescription point for a single beam in spine should be the anterior border of the vertebral body taken from imaging and is usually between 5 and 7 cm in the cervical and thoracic region and 7–8 cm in the lumbar region.
- The prescription point for opposing anterior and posterior beams is the MPD.
- The prescription point for electron therapy is 100 percent on the central axis and the energy is chosen to cover the target volume at depth by the 90% isodose. Orthovoltage beams are prescribed with D_{max} at 100% isodose line.

Doses

The 8 Gy single fraction or 20 Gy in 5 daily fractions of 4 Gy given in 1 week or 30 Gy in 10 daily fractions of 3 Gy given in 2 weeks. For hemibody EBRT: Lower 8 Gy single fraction and upper 6 Gy single fraction.

BRAIN METASTASES

- The most common primary site is the lung followed by breast.
- MRI is the standard of care for imaging.
- Sudden increase in cerebral edema or hemorrhage into a metastatic lesion can lead to the patient presenting with sudden loss of consciousness or motor power, seizures, vomiting and headache and in certain acute situations may even be life-threatening.

Treatment

- Immediate treatment started with use of anticonvulsants (in cases of seizures) and medical decompression with a corticosteroid regimen of 10 mg IV or oral bolus, followed by a 4–6 mg every 6 to 8 hours of dexamethasone before tapering.
- In asymptomatic patients with little peritumoral edema or mass effect, initial corticosteroids may be reserved until the first sign of neurologic symptoms.
- Prophylactic anticonvulsants may not be initiated in newly diagnosed brain tumor patients who have not experienced a seizure.
- After controlling the raised intracranial pressure due to edema, palliative treatment is started.
- Whole brain RT (WBRT) is the standard of care in patients with multiple brain metastasis and should be given soon after the diagnosis of brain metastasis.

- A total dose of 30 Gy in 10 fractions is the standard for most patients. Shorter courses may be given (20 Gy in 5 fractions) in certain chemotherapy refractory progressive disease cases, but avoided in chemo-naïve cases as these patients will experience radiotherapy late toxicities if they have longer survival.
- Surgical resection is reserved for lesions causing life-threatening complications like hydrocephalus or herniation requiring urgent surgical intervention, or those patients with good performance status.
- Radiosurgery (RS) can provide an alternative to conventional surgery in cases where patient may not be a craniotomy candidate due to tumor location in eloquent areas or existing medical contraindications.

BLEEDING OR PAIN FROM ADVANCED MALIGNANCIES

- Bleeding from a lesion on the vulva, vagina, or cervix or from advanced tumors of the breast, bladder, bronchus and other sites can be effectively palliated with radiotherapy. Simple fields like opposing AP-PA beams for treatment of the bronchus or bladder, or small tangential beams for breast tumors, are used. The size is chosen clinically as the smallest needed to palliate the bleeding effectively with the fewest side effects.
- Pressure dressings or vaginal packing, with hospitalization and bed rest and starting radiotherapy, are successful in most clinically emergent vaginal bleeds.
- Reduction of bleeding occurs often within 24 – 48 hours of the first treatment.
- The first or second radiation treatment is usually delivered to the whole pelvis using anterior and posterior fields. A field reduction is used for the third fraction.

- A dose of 10 Gy whole pelvic radiation therapy is an effective means of palliating vaginal bleeding due to advanced or recurrent gynecologic cancer.
- In other case, following dose fractionations can be used:
  - Single 8 Gy fraction.
  - 20 Gy in 5 daily fractions given in 1 week.
  - 30 Gy in 5 fractions given in 6 weeks (6 Gy once weekly).

CHAPTER 19

Radiation Therapy: Accompaniments and their Management

Indu Bansal

It is necessary to include a margin of normal tissue around the tumor to allow for uncertainties in daily set-up and internal tumor motion. These uncertainties can be caused by internal movement (for example, respiration and bladder filling) and movement of external skin marks relative to the tumor position. To spare normal tissues (such as skin or organs which radiation must pass through in order to treat the tumor), shaped radiation beams are aimed from several angles of exposure to intersect at the tumor, providing a much larger absorbed dose there than in the surrounding, healthy tissue. These major improvements in radiation technology have made it more precise. In spite of shaped fields, radiation like other cancer treatments can cause side effects.

Unfortunately, early and late toxicity limits the deliverable intensity of radiotherapy, and might affect the long-term health-related quality of life of the patient. Higher doses can cause varying side effects during treatment (acute side effects), in the months or years following treatment (long-term side effects), or after re-treatment (cumulative side effects). The nature, severity, and longevity of side effects depend on the organs that receive the radiation, the treatment itself (type of radiation, dose, fractionation, concurrent chemotherapy), and the patient.

Most side effects are predictable and expected. Side effects from radiation are usually limited to the area of the patient's body that is under treatment. One of the aims of modern radiation therapy is to reduce side effects to a minimum, and to help the patient to understand and to deal with those side effects which are unavoidable. The reactions often begin by the second or third week of treatment and may last for several weeks after the treatment is over. Different radiation side effects and ways to cope them are described here.

RADIATION DERMATITIS

Radiation therapy can cause skin changes in the treatment area. There may be redness, dryness, puffiness, itching or peeling of skin (dry or wet desquamation) in the treatment area. If moist desquamation happens it may lead to wet, sore, or infected skin. Skin changes may start a few weeks after beginning radiation therapy and may persist for few weeks or life-long after completion of radiation.

How to Manage

- The ink markings for radiation therapy should not be washed.
- Rubbing, scrubbing, or scratching in the treatment area should be avoided.
- Any creams, lotions, perfumes, fragrant oils in radiation area should not be used.
- Application of very hot or cold items on the treatment area should be avoided.
- A mild soap without any fragrance or deodorant during shower or bath with lukewarm water can be used.
- Skin should be patted dry with a soft towel and not rubbed.
- If any skin product has to be used, it should be applied at least 4 hours before the treatment session.
- Cotton clothes and bed sheets made of soft fabrics should be used.
- Tight and constricting clothes are best avoided.

- Any bandages, band aids, or adhesive tapes in the treatment area should be avoided.
- Sun exposure should be avoided for a year after radiation and a broad-brimmed hat, long-sleeved shirt, and long pants should be worn when out in sun.
- A sunscreen with an SPF of 30 or higher should be used even on cloudy days or when outside for just a few minutes.
- Shaving if done should be done by an electric razor and pre-shave lotion should not be used.
- Rectal area should be cleaned with a baby wipe or squirt of water from a spray bottle. Sitz baths may be done in case of reactions.
- Antibiotics should be prescribed in case of infection.
- The affected part should be exposed to fresh air as far as possible.
- In case of troublesome skin reactions gentian violet lotion, steroid creams, silver sulphadiazine ointment or radiation protectants as Radiaguard lotion may be applied. If there is superadded infection, then antibiotic creams as Mupirocin may be prescribed.
- Patients who are getting concurrent targeted agents during radiation as cetuximab may have more severe skin reactions and appropriate treatment instituted.
- Radiation treatment may have to be stopped temporarily in case of grade 4 skin reactions.

MUCOSITIS

Radiation therapy to the head or neck can cause problems such as mouth sores, dry mouth and throat (*xerostomia*), loss of taste, tooth decay, changes in taste, infection of gums, teeth, or tongue, jaw stiffness (ankyloglossia), bone changes and thickened saliva.

It occurs due to radiation damage to salivary glands mainly parotid glands, taste buds, mandible, etc. Some problems like mouth sores, may go away after treatment ends. Others, such as taste changes, may last for months or even years. Some problems, like dry mouth, may never go away.

How to Manage

- A dental check-up at least 2 weeks before starting radiation therapy to head and neck area should be done. Any loose tooth should be extracted at least 2 weeks before radiation starts.
- Dentures should be kept clean, fitted well and not worn for too long hours.
- No tooth extraction should be done at least one year after radiation to head and neck area.
- The patients should be taught to check their mouth themselves everyday to see for mouth sores, white patches, or infection.
- The mouth should be kept moist.
- It can be done by sipping water often during the day, sucking on ice chips, chewing sugar-free gum or sucking on sugar-free hard candy or by using a saliva substitute to help moisten the mouth.
- Patients should be advised to brush teeth, gums, and tongue after every meal and at bedtime.
- An extra-soft toothbrush should be used and the bristles should be made softer by running warm water over them just before brushing.
- A flouride toothpaste and a fluoride gel may be used.
- Mouthwashes that contain alcohol should be avoided.
- Mouth should be rinsed every 1 to 2 hours with a solution of 1/4 teaspoon baking soda and 1/8 teaspoon salt mixed in 1 cup of warm water.
- Appropriate antibiotics should be prescribed in case of bacterial infection as soon as indicated.
- Oral or intravenous fluconazole may be used or clotrimazole lozenges may be sucked in case of candidiasis. Clotrimazole mouth paint may be applied.
- In case of severe reactions, a mixture of boroglycerine with tablet dexamethasone and nystatin mixture can be applied over sore area.

- Jaw muscles exercises under supervision of physiotherapist should be done. Mouth should be opened and closed at least 20 times as much as the patient can safely do without causing pain. This exercise should be done at least 3 times a day to prevent ankyloglossia.

Diet Care during Radiation

- Foods that are easy to chew and swallow should be chosen.
- A straw may be used instead of drinking from a cup.
- Small bites may be taken, and liquids sipped with meals.
- Moist soft foods such as cooked cereals, mashed potatoes, and scrambled eggs should be eaten.
- More of liquid diet should be consumed or food should be softened with gravy, sauce, broth, yogurt, or other liquids.
- Foods that are warm or at room temperature should be consumed.
- All tobacco products, including cigarettes, pipes, cigars, and chewing tobacco are prohibited.
- Drinks that contain alcohol should be avoided.
- Hot and spicy, crunchy foods should be avoided.
- Fruits and juices that are high in acid such as tomatoes, oranges, lemons, and grapefruits should not be taken.

ESOPHAGITIS

Radiation therapy to the neck or chest can cause the lining of esophagus to become inflamed and sore leading to esophagitis. They may occur 2 to 3 weeks after starting radiation and last for 4 to 6 weeks after radiation therapy has finished.

How to Manage

- Foods may be cut, blended, or shredded to make them easier to eat.

- Moist soft foods such as cooked cereals, mashed potatoes, and scrambled eggs can be tried.
- Food may be softened with gravy, sauce, broth, yogurt, or other liquids.
- Cool drinks may be consumed more.
- A straw may be used to sip drinks.
- Foods that are cool or at room temperature can be consumed.
- Instead of eating 3 large meals each day, 5 or 6 small meals and snacks should be eaten.
- Foods and drinks that are high in calories and protein to maintain optimum weight should be consumed.
- Sitting upright and bending head slightly forward when eating or drinking helps. Patient should remain sitting or standing upright for at least 30 minutes after eating.
- Hot foods and drinks, spicy foods, foods and juices that are high in acid, such as tomatoes and oranges, sharp, crunchy foods such as potato or corn chips, all tobacco products, such as cigarettes, pipes, cigars, and chewing tobacco should be avoided.
- Drinks that contain alcohol should be avoided.
- Foods that are high in calories and protein and foods that are easy to swallow should be tried.
- Mucaine gel with disprin gargles before meals may help in relieving symptoms.
- Lidocaine viscous before food can be prescribed.
- Analgesics as tramadol, paracetamol or combination of both as per severity of pain will help in easing the symptoms.
- If the patient has dysphagia to both solids and liquids, then Ryle's tube or PEG tube feeding will help in maintaining the nutritional status of patient.

XEROSTOMIA (DRY MOUTH)

Radiation therapy that is delivered to the head and neck area may also result in xerostomia. The salivary glands and tear glands have a radiation tolerance of about 30 Gy in 2 Gy fractions, a dose which is exceeded by most radical head and neck cancer treatments.

Xerostomia is a chronic dry-mouth condition caused by damage to the salivary glands. It can have a negative effect on quality of life by greatly impairing a patient's ability to speak, chew, swallow, and taste.

How to Manage

- Water or other beverages should be handy during meals.
- Softer, more liquid foods help.
- Lips may be moistened with lip balm.
- Sweet or tart foods or beverages, such as lemonade may be consumed, to help mouth produce saliva.
- Sugar-free hard candy or Popsicles or sugar-free gum may be sucked to help produce more saliva.
- Soft and pureed foods that are easier to swallow may be used.
- Eat foods with sauces, gravies, and salad dressings to make them moist and easier to swallow.
- Water should be sipped every few minutes to make swallowing and talking easier.
- If the dry mouth problem is severe, then artificial saliva substitutes may be used.
- Medicines as amifostine, pilocarpine may be prescribed.
- Utmost care should be taken to keep the dose of radiation to the minimum to parotid and submandibular glands.

NAUSEA AND VOMITING

Nausea and vomiting can occur after radiation therapy to the stomach, small intestine, colon, or parts of the brain. The risk for nausea and vomiting depends on dose of radiation, treatment area, and whether chemotherapy is also being administered. It may occur 30 minutes to many hours after end of radiation therapy session.

How to Manage

- Bland, easy-to-digest foods and drinks that do not upset stomach should be consumed.
- Relaxation before treatment as doing activities which patient enjoys helps in preventing nausea as reading a book, listening to music, or other hobbies.
- Instead of eating 3 large meals each day patient should be advised to eat 5 or 6 small meals and snacks and to eat slowly and not to rush.
- A lemon may be sniffed or a small piece of candied ginger eaten to ease nausea.
- Warm or cool (not hot or cold) foods and drinks should be eaten.
- An antiemetic as ondansetron, granisetron or domperidone may be prescribed half to one hour before radiotherapy session.
- Now, palosetron and ramosetron hydrochloride tablets and injections are also available.
- Aprepitant capsules and dexamethasone may be added, if nausea and vomiting does not settle.

CHANGES IN SMELL OR TASTE

- If certain foods that were once enjoyed become unappealing, other nutritious foods may be used that are now more appetizing.
- Flavor may be enhanced with herbs, spices, sauces or marinades.
- If citrus does not bother then a squirt of lemon or lime may be used on foods to perk up flavor.
- If smell bothers, cold foods may be eaten, which give off fewer aromas.

ANOREXIA

Cancer treatments can wipe out many normal cells in the body, including some of those that line the gastrointestinal tract, thus causing nausea. Cells in the mouth and nose can also be affected, causing changes in smell and taste that can make eating less desirable. If a person stops eating healthy, regular meals, the immune system could be further weakened, making it that much harder to fight the cancer. Poor nutritional status can also lead to a loss of muscle mass and an electrolyte imbalance, adding to already existing feelings of weakness and fatigue.

How to Manage

- Smaller more frequent meals every few hours are preferable.
- Drinking liquids during or just before meals should be avoided.
- Healthy, solid food will provide the body with better nutrition.
- Foods and beverages that supply only *empty calories*—that is, calories that do not provide nutritional benefits, such as sweets, alcohol, salty snacks and soda are best avoided.
- Healthy snacks (yogurt, nuts, cheese sticks) should be carried when going out.
- Five or more servings of fruits and vegetables and whole (not processed) grains are beneficial.
- Meal and snacks time should be scheduled and things done to make this time as pleasant as possible.
- An appropriate number of calories per day as per weight and height should be taken. To maintain current weight, a rule of thumb is 15 calories per pound of weight, per day.
- Make sure that no more than 30% of daily caloric intake comes from fat.
- Foods high in protein, which helps the body repair damaged tissues and boosts immune system are better. Multiply body weight by 0.5 to 0.6 to calculate target protein intake in grams.
- A liquid or powdered nutritional supplement may be used.

DIARRHEA

Radiation therapy to the pelvis, stomach, and abdomen can cause diarrhea. It can occur at any time during radiation therapy due to radiation exposure to healthy cells in the large and small bowels.

How to Manage

- At least 8 to 12 cups of clear liquid per day should be taken.
- Rather than 3 large meals, 5 or 6 small meals and snacks are preferable.
- Foods that are easy on the stomach (which means foods that are low in fiber, fat, and lactose) are better.
- Instead of toilet paper, a baby wipe or squirt of water from a spray bottle may be used to clean rectal area after bowel movements. Sitz baths with lukewarm water and crystals of potassium permaganate can be used in case of anal sores.
- Milk and dairy foods, spicy foods, foods or drinks with caffeine, (such as regular coffee, black tea, soda, and chocolate), foods or drinks that cause gas (such as cooked dried beans, cabbage, broccoli, soy milk, and other soy products), high fiber foods (raw fruits and vegetables, whole wheat breads and cereals), fried or greasy foods are best avoided.
- BRAT diet (bananas, rice, apple sauce, and toast) helps in controlling diarrhea.
- Electral ORS powder, coconut water after every loose motion replenishes the salt and electrolyte loss.
- Antidiarrheal agents and antimotility agents as lomotil may be prescribed as per need.
- In case of dehydration intravenous fluids may be administerd.

URINARY AND BLADDER CHANGES

Radiation therapy can harm the healthy cells of the bladder wall and urinary tract, which can cause inflammation, ulcers, and infection. So, it can cause urinary and bladder problems, as:

- Burning or pain while urination
- Trouble in starting urination

- Frequency or urgency to urinate
- Cystitis, (inflammation) of urinary tract
- Incontinence, or inability to control the flow of urine from bladder, especially when coughing or sneezing
- Frequent need to get up during sleep to urinate
- Blood in urine
- Bladder spasms, which are like painful muscle cramps

These problems start 3 to 5 weeks after starting radiation therapy and last for 2 to 8 weeks after treatment is over.

How to Manage

- At least 6 to 8 cups of fluids each day should be consumed so that urine is clear to light yellow in color.
- Coffee, black tea, alcohol, spices, and all tobacco products should be avoided.
- Urine examination to rule out infection should be done and antibiotics taken accordingly.
- Bladder exercises to improve bladder control should be done under supervision of a therapist.
- Alkalizers as citralka or alkasol can be used to make the urine pH alkaline.
- Urinary analgesics as pyridium can help in dysuria.

HAIR LOSS

Epilation (hair loss) may occur on any hair bearing skin with doses above 1 Gy. It only occurs within the radiation fields. Hair loss may be permanent with a single dose of 10 Gy, but if the dose is fractionated, permanent hair loss may not occur until dose exceeds 45 Gy.

Radiation therapy can cause hair loss because it damages hair roots on the part of body being treated. Hair loss starts in the treatment area 2 to 3 days after first radiation therapy session. It takes about a week for all the hair in the treatment area to fall. The hair may grow back 3 to 6 months after treatment is over. The hair that grow back, may not look or feel the way it did before. It may be thinner, or curly instead of straight or it may be darker or lighter in color than before.

How to Manage

- Plan ahead whether to cut or shave the head. An electric razor can be used to prevent nicking.
- If the patient is conscious about hair loss they can be advised to wear a hat, turban, scarf, fancy bandanas or wig.
- The best time to select a comfortable wig is before radiation therapy begins or soon after it starts so that the wig matches the color and style of hair.
- A mild shampoo, such as a baby shampoo may be used to wash hair. The hair should be dried by patting (not rubbing) it with a soft towel.
- Curling irons, electric hair dryers, curlers, hair bands, clips, or hair sprays should not be used during radiation.
- Hair colors, perms, gels, oil, etc. are best avoided.

FATIGUE

Fatigue from radiation therapy can range from a mild to an extreme feeling of being tired. Many people describe fatigue as feeling weak, weary, worn out, heavy, or slow. It can happen due to anemia, anxiety, depression, infection, lack of activity or due to medicines. Fatigue is typically more severe two to four hours after treatment. It can last from 6 weeks to 12 months after last radiation therapy session.

How to Manage

- Normal activities during radiation therapy should not be restricted, but balance between normal activity and periods of rest should be maintained.

- Maintenance of good nutritious balance diet is most important to combat fatigue.
- At least 8 hours sleep each night is preferable. Planned 15–20 minutes of short naps also help.
- It is important to stay active, but prioritization of the activities that are most important should be done.
- Short exercises as 15 to 30 minutes walk, stretches or *Yoga* help.
- Work should be continued as much as the body permits.
- Others' help may be sought in routine chores.

SEXUAL AND FERTILITY CHANGES

Sexual and fertility changes can happen when people get radiation therapy to the pelvic area as vagina, uterus, or ovaries and for males after radiation to the testicles or prostate. Sexual dysfunction may be caused by one or more of the following: physical changes from cancer surgery, chemotherapy, hormonal therapy, or radiation therapy, hormone changes, fatigue, pain, nausea and vomiting, medications that can reduce libido, fear of recurrence of the cancer, stress, depression, anxiety, changes in self-image and unhappiness or embarrassment with physical changes.

It can cause hormone changes and loss of interest in or inability to have sex. It can also affect fertility during and after radiation therapy. A female may have pain or discomfort while having sex. She can have vaginal dryness, itching, burning or vaginal stenosis. Symptoms of menopause as hot flashes, vaginal dryness, amenorrhea or infertility can occur. Males may have impotence, erectile dysfunction and low sperm count. The patient should be told before-hand about these side effects and measures taken to prevent them.

How to Manage

- Menstrual history of young females should always be taken to ensure that she is not pregnant. Patients should be advised not to get pregnant while having radiation therapy.

- Fertility issues should always be discussed with the patient before starting radiation therapy. If the patient is desirous of child bearing, then every effort should be done to preserve the fertility, such as cryopreservation of semen or eggs.
- Hormone replacement therapy, vaginal moisturizers or lubricants, may be used to prevent vaginal dryness.
- Vaginal stenosis can be prevented by advicing patients to use a vaginal dilator. While having sex, a water- or mineral oil-based lubricant such as K-Y jelly may be used.
- Scrotal shields should be used during radiation and transposition of ovaries out of radiation field may be done.

LOW BLOOD COUNTS (MYELOSUPPRESSION)

Blood counts, or the number of blood cells in circulation, can be affected by radiation. Some patients describe a sense of tiredness and fatigue. It is advised to check blood counts at least once every week during the radiation treatments. Just ensure that hemoglobin is at least 10 gm%, total leukocyte count >4000/cumm and platelet count is at least 1 lakh during radiation. Proper antibiotics or growth factors should be prescribed as per need to combat infection.

RADIATION PNEUMONITIS

Radiation pneumonitis is the acute manifestation of radiation-induced lung disease (RILD) and is relatively common following radiotherapy for chest wall or intrathoracic malignancies. The acute phase typically occurs between 4 and 12 weeks following completion of radiotherapy course, although they may be seen as early as 1 week, especially in patients receiving high total dose and/or also having received chemotherapy. Symptoms typically include: cough, dyspnea (exertional or at rest), low-grade fever, chest discomfort, pleuritic chest pain.

It reflects acute response of the lung to radiation and occurs due to loss of type I pneumocytes, increased capillary permeability resulting in interstitial and alveolar edema and ingress of inflammatory cells into the alveolar spaces. When changes are seen in the non-irradiated lung an immune mediated lymphocytic alveolitis has been postulated as the underlying cause.

Chest X-ray changes are nonspecific, but confined to the irradiation port, with airspace opacities being most common. Pleural effusions or atelectasis are also sometimes seen. In cases of early or subtle radiation induced pneumonitis, areas of ground-glass opacity may be evident on CT despite a normal chest X-ray. CT will show ground-glass opacities and/or airspace consolidation, tree-in-bud appearances, ipsilateral pleural effusion or atelectasis.

How to Manage

Steroids and bronchodilators can reduce the severity of acute radiation pneumonitis. Depending on the degree of injury changes may be mild and spontaneously resolve or progress to adult respiratory distress syndrome (ARDS) with high rate of mortality.

LATE SIDE EFFECTS

Late side effects are those that first occur at least 6 months after radiation therapy is over. Late side effects are rare, but they do happen. They occur months to years after treatment and are generally limited to the area that has been treated. They are often due to damage of blood vessels and connective tissue cells. Many late effects are reduced by fractionating treatment into smaller parts.These side effects will depend on the part of body that was treated, the dose and length of radiation and if chemotherapy was administered before, during, or after radiation therapy.

Lymphedema

Lymphedema is a swelling in an arm or a leg caused by a build-up of lymph fluid. It can happen if lymph nodes were removed during surgery or damaged by radiation therapy. It can lead to swelling on the face, the arm or leg on the side where radiation was administered. Early signs of lymphedema should be noticed as pain or a sense of heaviness in arm or leg, a feeling of tightness in arm or leg, trouble in putting on shoes or rings or weakness in arm or leg.

How to Manage

- Be active. Exercises can help prevent and treat lymphedema.
- Proper care of arm or leg is very essential.
- Skin should be kept moisturized by applying lotion at least once a day.
- Sunburns should be avoided. Sunscreens with an SPF of 30 or higher may be used and long sleeves and long pants worn if in the sun.
- Gloves should be worn while gardening or cooking.
- Toe nails should be clipped straight across, fingernails filed, and cuticles should not be cut.
- Feet should be kept clean and dry, cotton socks worn.
- Cuts should be cleaned with soap and water and then antibacterial ointment applied.
- Extreme hot or cold, such as ice packs or heating pads are best avoided.
- Pressure on arm or leg should be avoided. For example, do not cross legs when sitting or carry purse on the side that had radiation.
- Loose clothes that do not have tight elastic cuffs or waistbands should be worn.
- Very hot water baths should be avoided.
- Any injections, blood pressure measurements should be avoided lifelong on the operated arm.
- If lymphedema occurs, then elastic stockings may be worn. In case of severe lymphedema, lympha press therapy is an option.

Joint Changes

Radiation therapy can cause scar tissue and weakness in the part of the body that was treated. This can lead to loss of motion in joints, such as jaw, shoulders, or hips. Joint problems can show up months or years after radiation therapy is over.

How to Manage

- Early signs of joint problems should be noted.
- Trouble in opening mouth wide.
- Pain while making certain movements, such as reaching over head or putting hand in a back pocket.
- A physical therapist's help should be sought. The therapist can give exercises to decrease pain, increase strength, and improve movement.

Cognitive Decline

Cognitive decline can occur months to years after radiation to brain. Radio-induced neurocognitive impairment evolves in a biphasic pattern: a subacute transient decline with a peak at four months, and a late delayed irreversible impairment of NCF several months or years after completion of WBRT.

Side effects can include memory loss, problems doing mathematics, movement problems, incontinence, trouble thinking, or personality changes. Cognitive decline was especially apparent in young children, between the ages of 5 to 11. Studies found, for example, that the IQ of 5-year-old children declined each year after treatment by several IQ points.

How to Manage

- Dose and field of radiation should be minimized as much as possible.

- Oligometastasis is best treated with surgery or stereotactic radiation and whole brain radiation delayed as far as possible.
- A physical, occupational, or speech therapist's help may be sought.
- Whole brain radiation might specifically impair hippocampus-related functions, leading to the concept of hippocampus avoidance during WBRT.
- In patients who show complete response to chemotherapy, every attempt should be made to reduce the dose and volume of radiation field.
- Specific care should be taken in designing radiation fields in case of a child.
- Medicines may be prescribed or surgery for radiation necrosis attempted to help relieve the symptoms.

Radiation Proctitis

Radiation can involve long-term effects on the rectum including bleeding, diarrhea and urgency and is associated with radiation therapy to pelvic organs. The incidence is related to the dose of radiation, area of exposure, method of delivery, and the use of cytoprotective agents. The doses generally delivered to the pelvis vary from 45 to 50 Gy for adjuvant or neoadjuvant treatment for prostate or anorectal malignancies; up to 90 Gy is considered the definitive therapy for gynecological malignancies.

- Usually <45 Gy cause very few side effects.
- Doses between 45 and 70 Gy, which is the dosage range for most treatments, cause more complications.
- Doses above 70 Gy cause significant and long-standing injury to the surrounding area.
- Incidence of radiation proctitis range from 2 to 39% depending upon the dose of radiation.
- IMRT leads to incidence rates from 1–9%
- Particle radiation therapy in the range of 1%.

- With brachytherapy alone risk is 8–13% and up to 21% when used in combination with other modalities.

Acute radiation proctitis is defined as an inflammatory process involving only the superficial mucosa that occurs almost immediately after the initiation of therapy or up to 3 months after the onset of therapy. Symptoms including diarrhea, nausea, cramps, tenesmus, urgency, mucus discharge, and minor bleeding will develop in up to 20% of patients necessitating an interruption in treatment.

Chronic radiation proctitis can begin early, even during the acute phase of radiation proctitis, but symptoms may not become apparent until months to years later after the cessation of therapy (median 8–12 months after the completion of therapy). Symptoms of chronic proctitis may include those of acute radiation proctitis but may further include severe bleeding, strictures, perforation, fistula, and bowel obstruction. The incidence of chronic radiation proctitis is estimated at 2–20%.

How to Manage

- Acute proctitis is usually self-limiting, in up to 20% patients.
- Short interruptions in treatment may improve symptoms.
- Hydration, antidiarrheals, and possibly steroid or 5-amino-salicylate enemas may help.
- Chronic proctitis can be managed by noninvasive treatments as anti-inflammatory agents, sucralfate, short-chain fatty acids, hyperbaric, oxygen, antioxidants.
- Invasive treatments as ablation by rectal instillation of 4% formalin solution or direct topical application of a 10% formalin solution might be required at times.
- YAG lasers may be useful in the treatment of radiation proctitis.
- Diverting loop colostomy, proctectomy, resection with reconstruction when the stricture is higher in the rectum or an

advancement flap (mucosa or skin) when the rectal stricture is in the anus are the surgical options.

- A newer chlorite-based anti-inflammatory agent which contains the active ingredient OXO-K993 and is administered intravenously, WF10, has recently been studied for the treatment of radiation-induced proctitis.

Hypothyroidism

Hypothyroidism (abnormally low levels of thyroid hormone) is one of the more frequently encountered late complications of radiation therapy in patients where the radiation field includes the neck. This may occur in up to one-third of patients receiving radiation therapy. It is important for patients who have received radiation therapy to be tested on a regular basis because signs and symptoms of hypothyroidism occur very late and are subtle.

How to Manage

- Thyroid examination should be part of annual physical examination.
- Thyroid function tests at least annually in patients who have received radiation to neck.
- Proper medicines started, if hypopthyroidism is detected.

Heart Disease

Radiation affects every component of the heart, ranging from subclinical histopathologic changes to overt clinical disease. Pericardial involvement is most common and includes asymptomatic pericardial effusion and constrictive pericarditis. The diseases involving the myocardium, valvular apparatus, and conduction system are often subclinical. When symptomatic, they are often the harbinger of more lethal, but treatable, radiation-induced coronary artery disease (CAD). Improvements in the modern radiation delivery systems have minimized irradiation of the heart.

Cardiac toxicity after radiation treatment depends on several factors including total radiation dose, dose of radiation fractions, amount and areas of the heart treated, presence of tumor in or next to the heart, chemotherapy drugs used—the anthracyclines greatly increase the risk, age, weight, blood pressure, and family history and smoking.

Possible symptoms of coronary artery disease are: Uncomfortable pressure, fullness, squeezing or pain in the center of the chest that lasts a few minutes, or goes away and comes back, pain that spreads to the shoulders, neck or arms, chest discomfort with lightheadedness, fainting, sweating, nausea or shortness of breath.

How to Manage

- Techniques to reduce cardiac exposure (e.g. respiratory gating, intensity modulated radiation therapy) may be used judiciously.
- Annual blood pressure monitoring for patients who have received thoracic radiation.
- Baseline stress test and echocardiogram should be done.

Second Cancers

Advances in radiation therapy and chemotherapy have increased the chances of survival for many people with cancer today. Of all the possible late complications of cancer treatment, developing a second cancer is one of the most serious. Radiation as a potential cause of secondary malignancies is seen in a very small minority of patients—usually less than 1/1000. It usually occurs 20–30 years following treatment, although some hematological malignancies may develop within 5–10 years. In the vast majority of cases, this risk is greatly outweighed by the reduction in risk conferred by treating the primary cancer. The cancer occurs within the treated area of the patient.

How to Manage

- The most important aspect of treatment of secondary cancer is early diagnosis.
- Proper skin examination to rule out skin cancers.
- Monthly self-breast examination and yearly physical examination by a clinician for women who have received axillary or chest wall radiation.
- Women with Hodgkin's disease should begin mammography screening at an earlier age than the general population and this should be done annually for life.
- Breast MRI in addition to mammogram in women who received radiation between 10 and 30 years of age.
- Also, men and women who are cancer survivors should undergo screening for bowel cancer at an earlier age than the general population and also continue it for life.
- Usually, cancers of a certain type are treated the same regardless of whether they are primary or secondary.

CHAPTER 20

Teletherapy Machines and Other Instruments

Kanika Sharma

LINEAR ACCELERATOR (FIGS 20.1 TO 20.4)

The first linear accelerator became operational in 1953 at the Radiation Research Center of the Medical Research Council at Hammersmith Hospital in London.

It is a device that uses high-frequency electromagnetic waves to accelerate charged particles such as electrons to high energies through a linear tube. The high-energy electron beam itself can be used for treating superficial tumors, or it can be made to strike a target to produce X-rays for treating deep-seated tumors.

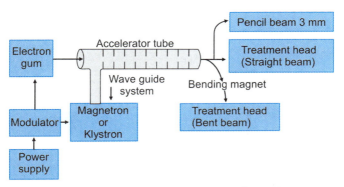

Fig. 20.1 Typical medical linear accelerator

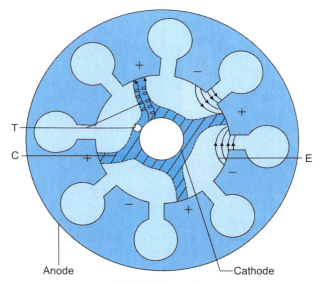

Fig. 20.2 Magnetron

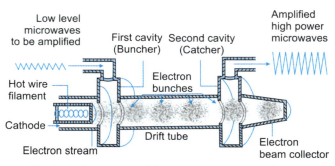

Fig. 20.3 Cross-sectional drawing of a two-cavity Klystron

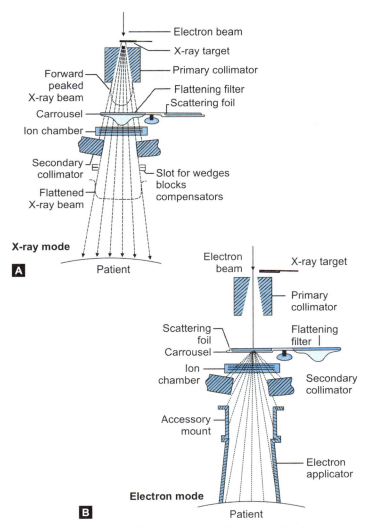

Figs 20.4A and B Components of treatment head

The electrons are accelerated either by traveling or stationary electromagnetic waves.

- The standing wave structures provide maximum reflection of the waves at both ends of the structure so that the combination of forward and reverse traveling waves will give rise to stationary waves.
- In the standing wave design, the microwave power is coupled into the structure via side coupling cavities rather than through the beam aperture.

A power supply provides direct current power to the modulator, which includes the pulse-forming network and a switch tube known as hydrogen thyratron. These pulses are delivered to the magnetron or klystron and simultaneously to the electron gun.

Pulsed microwaves produced in the magnetron or klystron are injected into the accelerator tube or structure via a waveguide system. At the proper instant electrons, produced by an electron gun, are also pulse injected into the accelerator structure.

The accelerator structure waveguide consists of a copper tube with its interior divided by copper discs or diaphragms of varying aperture and spacing. It is evacuated to a high vacuum. As the electrons are injected into the accelerator structure they interact with the electromagnetic field of the microwaves. The electrons gain energy from the sinusoidal electric field by an acceleration process.

As the high-energy electrons emerge from the exit window of the accelerator structure, they are in the form of a pencil beam (about 3 mm in diameter).

In the low-energy linacs (4–6 MV) with relatively short accelerator tube, the electrons are allowed to proceed straight on and strike a target for X-ray production. In the higher-energy linacs (15–18 MV), the accelerator structure is long and, therefore, is placed horizontally or at an angle with respect to the horizontal. The electrons are then bent through an angle (usually about 90 or 270 degrees) between the accelerator structure and the target.

Magnetron

It is a high-power oscillator, generating microwave pulses of several microseconds duration and with a repetition rate of several hundred pulses per second. The frequency of the microwaves within each pulse is about 3,000 MHz.

It is cylindrical, having a central cathode and an outer anode with resonant cavities. The space between the cathode and the anode is evacuated. The cathode is heated by an inner filament and the electrons are generated by thermionic emission. A static magnetic field is applied perpendicular to the plane of the cross-section of the cavities and a pulsed DC electric field is applied between the cathode and the anode. Under the simultaneous influence of the magnetic field, the electrons move in complex spirals toward the resonant cavities, radiating energy in the form of microwaves.

Klystron

The klystron is a microwave amplifier. The electrons produced by the cathode are accelerated into the first cavity, called the buncher cavity. The microwaves set up an alternating electric field across the cavity. The velocity of the electrons is altered by the action of this electric field. Some electrons are speeded up while others are slowed down and some are unaffected. This results in bunching of electrons. As the electron bunches arrive at the catcher cavity, they induce charges on the ends of the cavity and thereby generate a retarding electric field. The electrons suffer deceleration, and the kinetic energy of electrons is converted into high-power microwaves.

Linac X-ray Beam

Bremsstrahlung X-rays are produced when the electrons are incident on a target of a high-Z material such as tungsten. The target is water cooled and is thick enough to absorb most of the incident electrons. The electron energy is converted into a spectrum of X-ray.

Treatment Head

The treatment head consists of a thick shell of high-density shielding material such as lead, tungsten, or lead-tungsten alloy. It contains an X-ray target, scattering foil, flattening filter, ion chamber, fixed and movable collimator, and light localizer system.

Target and Flattening Filter

To make the beam intensity uniform across the field, a flattening filter is inserted in the beam. This filter is usually made of lead, although tungsten, uranium, steel, aluminum have been used.

Beam Collimation and Monitoring

The treatment beam is first collimated by a fixed primary collimator located immediately beyond the X-ray target. In the case of X-rays, the collimated beam then passes through the flattening filter. In the electron mode, the filter is moved out of the way.

The flattened X-ray beam or the electron beam is incident on the dose monitoring chambers. The monitoring system consists of several ion chambers or a single chamber with multiple plates.

After passing through the ion chambers, the beam is further collimated by a continuously movable X-ray collimator. This collimator consists of two pairs of lead or tungsten blocks (jaws) which provide a rectangular opening from 0×0 to the maximum field size (40×40 cm) projected at a standard distance such as 100 cm from the X-ray source.

The field size definition is provided by a light localizing system in the treatment head. A combination of mirror and a light source located in the space between the chambers and the jaws projects a light beam as if emitting from the X-ray focal spot.

Gantry

The source of radiation can rotate about a horizontal axis. As the gantry rotates, the collimator axis coincident moves in a vertical plane. The point of intersection of the collimator axis and the axis of rotation of the gantry is known as the isocenter.

The linear accelerator can also be used in stereotactic radiosurgery similar to that achieved using the gamma knife on targets within the brain. It delivers a uniform dose of high-energy X-ray to the region of the patient's tumor. A linear accelerator is also used for Intensity-Modulated Radiation Therapy (IMRT).

CYBERKNIFE

The **CyberKnife** is a frameless robotic radiosurgery system invented by John R Adler, a Stanford University Professor of Neurosurgery and Radiation Oncology. The two main elements of the CyberKnife are (1) the radiation produced from a small linear particle accelerator and (2) a robotic arm which allows the energy to be directed at any part of the body from any direction.

The CyberKnife system is a method of delivering radiotherapy, with the intention of targeting treatment more accurately than standard radiotherapy. It is not widely available, although the number of centers offering the treatment around the world has grown in recent years to over 150, particularly centered in the USA, Japan, the Far East, India and Europe.

GAMMA KNIFE

A **gamma knife** (or **Leksell gamma knife**) is a device used to treat brain tumors with a high dose of radiation therapy in one day. The gamma knife device contains 201 cobalt-60 sources of approximately 30 curies (1.1 TBq) each, placed in a circular array in a heavily shielded assembly. The device aims gamma radiation through a target point in the patient's brain. The patient wears a specialized helmet that is surgically fixed to his skull so that the brain tumor remains stationary at target point of the gamma rays. An ablative dose of radiation is thereby sent through the tumor in one treatment session, while surrounding brain tissues are relatively spared.

TELECOBALT MACHINE (FIG. 20.5)

Of all the radionuclides, ^{60}Co has proved to be the most suitable for external beam radiotherapy. The reasons for its choice over radium and cesium are higher possible specific activity, greater radiation output per curie and higher average photon energy. In addition, radium is much more expensive and has greater self-absorption of its radiation than either cesium or cobalt.

The ^{60}Co source is produced by irradiating ordinary stable ^{59}Co with neutrons in a reactor. It is usually in the form of a solid cylinder, discs, or pellets, is contained inside a stainless-steel capsule and sealed by welding. This capsule is placed into another steel capsule which is again sealed by welding. The double-welded seal is necessary to prevent any leakage of the radioactive material.

The ^{60}Co source decays to ^{60}Ni with the emission of β particles (E_{max} = 0.32 MeV) and two photons per disintegration of energies 1.17 and 1.33 MeV. These rays constitute the useful treatment beam. The β particles are absorbed in the cobalt metal and the stainless-steel capsules resulting in the emission of Bremsstrahlung X-rays and a small amount of characteristic X-rays. The other contaminants to the treatment beam are the lower-energy β rays produced by the interaction of the primary β radiation with the source itself, the surrounding capsule, the source housing, and the collimator system.

Modern isocentric ^{60}Co teletherapy machines have a source-to-axis distance of 80–100 cm. Source activities vary from about 5,000–13,000 Ci in 1.5–2.0 cm diameter sources, and yield exposure rates of 150–250 R/min at 1 meter.

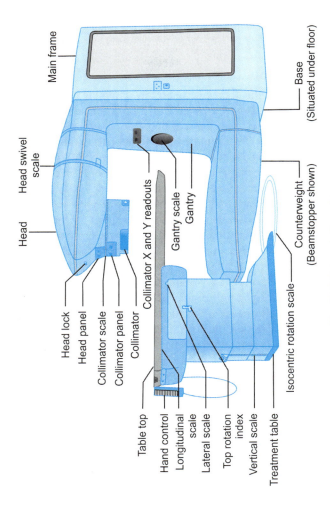

Fig. 20.5 Tele-cobalt machine

Maximum field sizes of 40×40 cm at the machine isocenter are available on newer machines. The radiation consists of 1.17 and 1.33 MeV with an average of 1.25 MeV γ-rays having a $d_{1/2}$ in tissue of about 10 cm.

Source Housing

The housing for the source is called the source head. The source head consists of a steel shell filled with lead for shielding purposes and a device for bringing the source in front of an opening in the head from which the useful beam emerges. Also, a heavy metal alloy sleeve is provided to form an additional primary shield when the source is in the off position. A typical teletherapy ^{60}Co source is a cylinder of diameter ranging from 1.0 to 2.0 cm and is positioned in the cobalt unit with its circular end facing the patient.

A number of methods have been developed for moving the source from the off position to the on position. These include: (a) the source mounted on a rotating wheel inside the source-head to carry the source from the off position to the on position; (b) the source mounted on a heavy metal drawer plus its ability to slide horizontally through a hole running through the source-head in the on position the source faces the aperture for the treatment beam and in the off position the source moves to its shielded location and a light source mounted on the same drawer occupies the on position of the source; (c) mercury is allowed to flow into the space immediately below the source to shut off the beam; and (d) the source is fixed in front of the aperture and the beam can be turned on and off by a shutter consisting of heavy metal jaws.

Beam Collimation and Penumbra

A collimator system is designed to vary the size and shape of the beam. The simplest form of a continuously adjustable diaphragm consists of two pairs of heavy metal blocks. Each pair can be moved independently to obtain a square or a rectangle-shaped field.

Some collimators are multi-vane type, i.e. multiple blocks to control the size of the beam. The inner surface of the blocks is made parallel to the central axis of the beam, the radiation will pass through the edges of the collimating blocks resulting in what is known as the transmission penumbra. The extent of this penumbra will be more pronounced for larger collimator openings because of greater obliquity of the rays at the edges of the blocks. This effect has been minimized in some designs by shaping the collimator blocks so that the inner surface of the blocks remains always parallel to the edge of the beam. In these collimators, the blocks are hinged to the top of the collimator housing so that the slope of the blocks is coincident with the included angle of the beam.

CYCLOTRON (FIG. 20.6)

The cyclotron accelerates heavy charged particles such as protons, deutrons, and heavy ions using a high-frequency, alternating voltage (potential difference) applied across two conducting

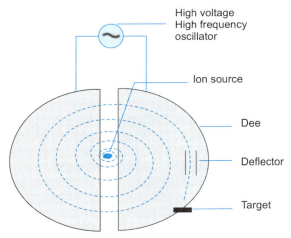

Fig. 20.6 The principle of operation of a cyclotron

D-shaped evacuated half-cylinders (Ds). A fixed magnetic field, perpendicular to the top of the two Ds, forces the charged particles to travel in a circular path. The charged particles accelerate only when passing through the gap between the two Ds. The beam spirals out to the edge of the container as the particles' speeds increase. At this point, the particles' speed approaches the speed of light. Proton beam energies of 200–250 MeV is considered adequate for most radiation therapy applications. Beam spreading is accomplished by passive modulation (scattering foils) or dynamic pencil beam-scanning systems.

SYNCHROCYCLOTRON/SYNCHROTRON

A synchrocyclotron varies either the magnetic field or the frequency of electric field; a synchrotron varies both. By increasing these features as the particles gain energy, their path can be held constant as they are accelerated. This allows the vacuum container for the particles to be a large, thin torus.

BETATRON (FIG. 20.7)

The operation is based on the principle that an electron in a changing magnetic field experiences acceleration in a circular

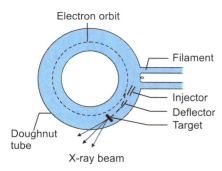

Fig. 20.7 The operation of a betatron

orbit. The accelerating tube is shaped like a hollow doughnut and is placed between the poles of an alternating current magnet. A pulse of electrons is introduced into this evacuated doughnut by an injector at the moment an alternating current cycle begins. As the magnetic field rises, electrons experience acceleration continuously and spin with increasing velocity around the tube. By the end of the first quarter cycle of the alternating magnetic field, the electrons have made several thousand revolutions and achieved maximum energy. At this instant or earlier, depending on the energy required, the electrons are then made to spiral out of the orbit by an additional attractive force. The high-energy electrons then strike a target to produce X-rays or a scattering foil to produce a broad beam of electrons. The X-ray dose rates and field size capabilities of medical betatrons are low compared with medical linacs and even modern cobalt units. But in the electron therapy mode, the beam current is adequate to provide a high dose rate.

TRANSFORMER UNITS

Resonant transformer units have been used to generate X-rays from 300–2,000 kV. The secondary of the high-voltage transformer is connected in parallel with capacitors inside the X-ray tube. This combination of transformer secondary and the capacitance in parallel exhibits the phenomenon of resonance. At the resonant frequency, the oscillating potential attains very high amplitude. Thus the peak voltage across the X-ray tube becomes very large when the transformer is tuned to resonate at the input frequency. Since the electrons attain high energies before striking the target, a transmission-type target may be used to obtain the X-ray beam on the other side of the target.

VAN DE GRAAFF GENERATOR (FIG. 20.8)

The Van de Graaff machine is an electrostatic accelerator designed to accelerate charged particles. In radiotherapy, the unit accelerates

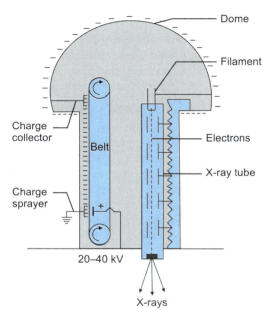

Fig. 20.8 Van de Graaff generator

electrons to produce high-energy X-rays, typically at 2 MV and capable of producing energies up to 10 MV. In this machine, a charge voltage of 20–40 kV is applied across a moving belt of insulating material. A corona discharge takes place and electrons are sprayed onto the belt, from where they are carried to the top and are removed by a collector connected to a spherical dome. As the negative charges collect on the sphere, a high potential is developed between the sphere and the ground. This potential is applied across the X-ray tube consisting of a filament, a series of metal rings, and a target. The rings are connected to resistors to provide a uniform drop of potential from the bottom to the top. X-rays are produced when the electrons strike the target.

RADIOISOTOPES

A radionuclide is an atom with an unstable nucleus, characterized by excess energy which is available to be imparted either to a newly-created radiation particle within the nucleus, or else to an atomic electron. The radionuclide, in this process, undergoes radioactive decay, and emits a gamma ray(s) and/or subatomic particles. Radionuclides may occur naturally, but can also be artificially produced.

Artificially produced radionuclides can be produced by nuclear reactors, particle accelerators or by radionuclide generators:

Radioisotopes produced with nuclear reactors use the high flux of neutrons present. The neutrons activate elements placed within the reactor. A typical product from a nuclear reactor is thallium-201 and iridium-192.

Particle accelerators such as cyclotrons accelerate particles to bombard a target to produce radionuclides. Cyclotrons accelerate protons at a target to produce positron emitting radioisotopes, e.g. fluorine-18. Radionuclide generators contain a parent isotope that decays to produce a radioisotope. The parent is usually produced in a nuclear reactor. Example is the technetium-99m. Trace radionuclides are those that occur in tiny amounts in nature.

The physical properties of radioisotopes shown in **Tables 21.1 and 21.2**.

Radium

- Produced by disintegration of $^{230}U_{90}$.
- Half-life-1626 years.
- Decays to produce radon by emission of alpha particle and γ-ray of 0.18 MeV energy.
- Radon further decays to daughter products. With release of 72 different energies. Maximum γ-ray energy is 2.4 MeV.
- Source comes with iridium platinum alloy wall of thickness of 0.5–1 mm.
- It is in form of a powder of radium sulfate mixed with barium sulfate.

Table 20.1 Physical properties of radioisotopes

Property	Palladium 103	Americium 241	Samarium 145	Ytterbium 169	Strontium 90	Yttrium 90
Half-life	17d	432 y	340 d	32 d	28.9 y	64 h
Average energy MeV	.02–.497	.013–.06	.038–.061	.049–.308		
Mean energy MeV	.021	.06	.41	.093	2.24	2.27
Beta energy max						
HVT in lead (mm)	.008	.125	.06	.2		
TVT in lead (mm)	.03	.4	.2	.7		
Gamma ray constant $Rh^{-1} mCi^{-1} cm^2$						
Exposure ray constant $Rh^{-1} mCi^{-1} cm^2$	1.48	.112	.885	1.8		
Air Kerma rate constant $\mu Gy\ h^{-1}\ MBq^{-1}\ m^2$	.035	.0029	.021	.0425		

Table 20.2 Physical properties of radioisotopes

Property	Cobalt 60	Iodine 125	Cesium 137	Tantalum 182	Iridium 192	Gold 198	Radon 222	Radium 226
Half-life	5.26 yr	60.1 d	30 y	115 d	74.2 d	2.7 d	3.82 d	1600 y
Average energy (MeV)	1.17–1.33	0.027–0.035	0.662	0.043–1.453	0.136–1.062	0.412–1.088	0.047–2.44	0.047–2.44
Mean (MeV)	1.25	.0029	.662	.67	.38	.416	.83	.83
Beta energy (Max)	.313	.0025	1.17	.51	.67	.96	3.26	3.26
HVT in lead (mm)	11	.1	6	12	3	3	14	14
TVT in lead (mm)	46	.004–.05	22	39	12	11	42	42
Gamma ray constant $Rh^{-1} mCi^{-1} cm^2$	13.07		3.23	6.71	4.62	2.32	2.32	9.068
Exposure ray constant $Rh^{-1} mCi^{-1} cm^2$	13.07	1.45	3.28	7.75	4.69	2.34	10.27	10.15
Air Kerma rate constant $uGy\ h^{-1} MBq^{-1} m^2$	.3064	.034	.077	.183	.111	.056	.1971	.1971

Cesium 137

- It is a fission product of uranium in nuclear reactor.
- Half-life – 30 years.
- Maximum photon energy–0.662 MeV.
- Source is in form of powder sealed by iridium-platinum alloy. It is available as tubes, needles and spheres.

Cobalt 60

- It is a radium substitute.
- Half-life 5.26 years.
- Produced by n-γ reaction in reactors from stable cobalt.
- It decays by β-emission to form stable nickel.
- Average photon energy is 1.25 MeV.

Iridium 192

Produced by n-γ reaction in reactors from Ir 191.

Half-life is 74.2 days.

Decays by β emission and electron capture to platinum and osmium. The excited daughter nuclei emit β- and γ-rays. It is available in form of:

- Flexible wires (0.5 or 0.3 mm).
  Each wire is an active platinum-iridium core encapsulated in 0.5 mm platinum sheath.
- Hair pins or single pins.
- Seeds preloaded on nylon tubes (like ribbons).
- Capsules (5.5 mm × .5 mm) as afterloading sources for HDR.

Phosphorus 32

An isotope of phosphorus half-life is 14 days, mode of decay: beta to S-32.

Phosphorus-32 is useful in the identification of malignant tumors because cancerous cells tend to accumulate phosphates more than normal cells do.

For many years, ^{32}P-chromic phosphate (32P-CP) intraperitoneal instillations and platinum analogue chemotherapy have been used to treat disseminated ovarian cancer. Phosphorus-32 CP low-dose intraperitoneal treatments in conjunction with platinum analogue chemotherapy is a promising approach for the treatment of disseminated intraperitoneal ovarian cancer.

Strontium 90

- A radioactive isotope of strontium.
- Half-life of 28.8 years.
- It is a product of nuclear fission. It is a pure beta emitter.

^{90}Sr undergoes β-decay with decay energy of 0.546 MeV to an electron and the yttrium isotope 90Y, which in turn, undergoes β-decay with half-life of 64 hours and decay energy 2.28 MeV for beta particles to an electron and 90Zr (zirconium), which is stable.

90Sr and 89Sr can be used in treatment of bone cancer. Strontium-90 exhibits biochemical behavior similar to calcium, the next lighter Group 2 element. After entering the organism, most often by ingestion with contaminated food or water, about 70–80% of the dose gets excreted. Virtually all remaining strontium-90 is deposited in bones and bone marrow, with the remaining 1% remaining in blood and soft tissues. Its presence in bones can cause bone cancer, cancer of nearby tissues.

INSTRUMENTS

Film Badge (Fig. 20.9)

Personnel dosimetry film badges are commonly used to measure and record radiation exposure due to gamma rays, X-rays and beta particles. The badge consists of two parts: photographic film, and a holder. The film is packaged in a light proof, vapor proof envelope preventing light, moisture or chemical vapors from affecting the film.

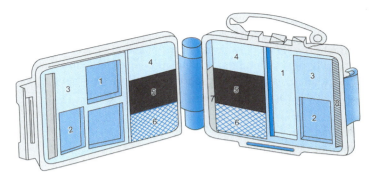

Fig. 20.9 Film badge holder: A photographic film with a fast emulsion on the one side and slow emulsion on the other is enclosed in the holder for monitoring radiation exposure. The radiation is measured by the degree of blackening of the film. The holder incorporates several filters for measuring different types of radiation. Beta dose is measured in the open window; gamma under the Pb; thermal neutrons by taking the difference between Pb + Cd and Pb + Sn filters. The 300 mg/cm² and 50 mg/cm² filters allow corrections for the beta and low energy gamma doses. The lead edge shielding minimizes edge effects at the boundary of the various filters. Indium foil is for criticality accidents. 1. Open window (β dose); 2. 50 mg/cm² plastic (low energy γ rays); 3. 300 mg/cm² plastics; 4. 0.004" dural; 5. 0.028 Cd 0.012" Pb; 6. 0.028 Sn 0.012" Pb; 7. 0.012"Pb edge shielding; 8. 0.4 gm of indium

The film is removed and developed to measure exposure.

The film is sensitive to radiation and, once developed, exposed areas increase in optical density (i.e. blacken) in response to incident radiation. One badge may contain several films of different sensitivities or, more usually, a single film with multiple emulsion coatings. The film is coated with two different emulsions. One side is coated with a large grain, fast emulsion that is sensitive to low levels of exposure. The other side of the film is coated with a fine grain, slow emulsion that is less sensitive to exposure. If the radiation exposure causes the fast emulsion in the processed film to be darkened to a degree that it cannot be interpreted, the fast emulsion is removed and the dose is computed using the slow emulsion.

Holder: The holder may contain a number of filters that attenuate certain types of radiation, such that only the target radiation is monitored. To monitor gamma rays or X-rays, the filters are metal, usually tin or lead. To monitor beta particle emission, the filters use various densities of plastic. The series of filters to determine the quality of the radiation. Radiation of a given energy is attenuated to a different extent by various types of absorbers. Therefore, the same quantity of radiation incident on the badge will produce a different degree of darkening under each filter. By comparing these results, the energy of the radiation can be determined and the dose can be calculated knowing the film response for that energy. The badge holder also contains an open window to determine radiation exposure due to beta particles. Beta particles are effectively shielded by a thin amount of material.

The badge is typically worn on the outside of clothing, around the chest or torso.

Advantages

The film badge has several advantages over other types of dosimetry:

- *Permanent record of exposure:* The developed film is physical evidence of the radiation exposure. The film can be stored after developing and reading, and could be reviewed at a later date if there is a query over exposure.
- *Exposure pattern discrimination:* A film badge offers limited discrimination between different patterns of exposure. A single exposure tends to leave sharp shadows on the film from the filters, whereas multiple small exposures at different angles will leave a rim of blurring around the filters. This may allow the linking of a dose with a specific incident and provides a degree of protection against tampering (e.g. deliberate exposure to a radiation source).

- *Radiation type detection:* Use of multiple filters allows separate measurement of beta and gamma exposure, and estimation of energy spectra. Additional filters can be added to detect neutron radiation (e.g. cadmium). The sensitivity of film to low energy (< 20 keV) gamma or X-radiation can be better than electronic dosimeters.

     It is quite accurate for exposures greater than 100 millirem.

     Disadvantages are that it must be developed and read by a processor (which is time consuming), prolonged heat exposure can affect the film, and exposures of less than 20 millirem of gamma radiation cannot be accurately measured.

TLD Badge

Used for Personal Dosimetry

Thermoluminescent dosimeters (TLD) are often used instead of the film badge. It is worn for a period of time (usually 3 months or less) and then must be processed to determine the dose received, if any.

   Thermoluminescent dosimeters can measure doses as low as 1 millirem, but under routine conditions their low-dose capability is approximately the same as for film badges. TLDs have a precision of approximately 15% for low doses. This precision improves to approximately 3% for high doses.

   A TLD is a phosphor, such as lithium fluoride (LiF) or calcium fluoride (CaF), in a solid crystal structure. When a TLD is exposed to ionizing radiation at ambient temperatures, the radiation interacts with the phosphor crystal and deposits all or part of the incident energy in that material. Some of the atoms in the material that absorb that energy become ionized, producing free electrons and areas lacking one or more electrons, called holes. Imperfections in the crystal lattice structure act as sites where free electrons can become trapped and locked into place.

   Heating the crystal causes the crystal lattice to vibrate, releasing the trapped electrons in the process. Released electrons return to the original ground state, releasing the captured energy from ionization as light, hence the name thermoluminescent. Released light is counted using photomultiplier tubes and the number of photons counted is proportional to the quantity of radiation striking the phosphor.

Instead of reading the optical density (blackness) of a film, as is done with film badges, the amount of light released versus the heating of the individual pieces of thermoluminescent material is measured. The "glow curve" produced by this process is then related to the radiation exposure. The process can be repeated many times.

The advantages of a TLD over other personnel monitors are its linearity of response to dose, its relative energy independence, and its sensitivity to low doses. It is also reusable, which is an advantage over film badges. However, no permanent record or re-readability is provided and an immediate, on the job readout is not possible.

Pocket Dosimeter

Pocket dosimeters are used to provide an immediate reading of exposure to X-rays and gamma rays. The two types commonly used in industrial radiography are the Direct Read Pocket Dosimeter and the Digital Electronic Dosimeter.

Direct Read Pocket Dosimeter (Fig. 20.10)

A direct reading pocket ionization dosimeter is generally of the size and shape of a fountain pen. The dosimeter contains a small ionization chamber with a volume of approximately two milliliters.

Inside the ionization chamber is a central wire anode, and attached to this wire anode is a metal coated quartz fiber. Electrostatic repulsion deflects the quartz fiber, and the greater the charge, the greater the deflection of the quartz fiber.

Radiation incident on the chamber produces ionization inside the active volume of the chamber. The electrons produced by ionization are attracted to, and collected by, the positively charged central

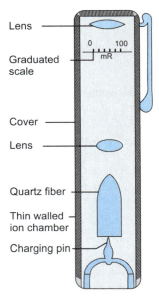

Fig. 20.10 Pen-type quartz fiber pocket dosimeter

anode. This collection of electrons reduces the net positive charge and allows the quartz fiber to return in the direction of the original position. The amount of movement is directly proportional to the amount of ionization which occurs.

By pointing the instrument at a light source, the position of the fiber may be observed through a system of built-in lenses. The fiber is viewed on a translucent scale which is graduated in units of exposure. Typical dosimeters have a full scale reading of 200 milliroentgens.

Advantage of a pocket dosimeter is its ability to provide an immediate reading of radiation exposure. It also has the advantage of being reusable.

Disadvantages: The limited range, inability to provide a permanent record, and the potential for discharging and reading loss due to dropping or bumping,

The dosimeters must be recharged and recorded at the start of each working shift. Charge leakage, or drift, can also affect the reading of a dosimeter. Leakage should be no greater than 2% of full scale in a 24 hour period.

Digital Electronic Dosimeter

These dosimeters record dose information and dose rate. These dosimeters most often use Geiger-Müller counters. The output of the radiation detector is collected and, when a predetermined exposure has been reached, the collected charge is discharged to trigger an electronic counter. The counter then displays the accumulated exposure and dose rate in digital form.

Survey Meters

They are used for area monitoring.

There are many different models of survey meters available to measure radiation in the field. They all basically consist of a detector and a readout display. Analog and digital displays are available. Most of the survey meters used for industrial radiography use a gas filled detector.

Gas filled detectors consist of a gas filled cylinder with two electrodes. Sometimes, the cylinder itself acts as one electrode, and a needle or thin taut wire along the axis of the cylinder acts as the other electrode. A voltage is applied to the device so that the central needle or wire becomes an anode and the other electrode or cylinder wall becomes the cathode. The gas becomes ionized whenever the counter is brought near radioactive substances. The electric field created by the potential difference between the anode and cathode causes the electrons of each ion pair to move to the anode while the positively charged gas atom is drawn to the cathode. This results in an electrical signal that is amplified correlated to exposure and displayed as a value.

Depending on the voltage applied between the anode and the cathode, the detector may be considered an ion chamber, a proportional counter, or a Geiger-Müller (GM) detector.

Ion Chamber Counter

Ion chambers have a relatively low voltage between the anode and cathode, which results in a collection of only the charges produced in the initial ionization event. This type of detector produces a weak output signal that corresponds to the number of ionization events. Higher energies and intensities of radiation will produce more ionization, which will result in a stronger output voltage.

Collection of only primary ions provides information on true radiation exposure. An ion chamber survey meter is used in the field when performing gamma radiography because it will provide accurate exposure measurements regardless of the radioactive isotope being used.

Proportional Counter

Proportional counter detectors use a slightly higher voltage between the anode and cathode. Due to the strong electrical field, the charges produced in the initial ionization are accelerated fast enough to ionize other electrons in the gas. The electrons produced in these secondary ion pairs, along with the primary electrons, continue to gain energy as they move towards the anode, and as they do, they produce more and more ionizations. The result is that each electron from a primary ion pair produces a cascade of ion pairs. This effect is known as gas multiplication or amplification. In this voltage regime, the number of particles liberated by secondary interactions is proportional to the number of ions produced by the passing ionizing particle. Like ion chamber detectors, proportional detectors discriminate between types of radiation. However, they require very stable electronics which are expensive and fragile. Proportional detectors are usually only used in a laboratory setting.

Geiger-Müller Counter

Geiger-Müller (GM) counters operate under even higher voltages between the anode and the cathode (usually in the 800–1200 volt range). The high voltage accelerates the charges produced in the initial ionization to where they have enough energy to ionize other electrons in the gas. However, this cascading of ion pairs occurs to a much larger degree and continues until the counter is saturated with ions. This occurs in a fraction of a second and results in an electrical current pulse of constant voltage. The collection of the large number of secondary ions in the GM region is known as an avalanche and produces a large voltage pulse.

The electronic circuit of a GM counters counts and records the number of pulses and the information is often displayed in counts per minute. When the volume of gas in the chamber is completely ionized, ion collection stops until the electrical pulse discharges.

Due to their ability to display individual ionizing events, GM counters are generally more sensitive to low levels of radiation than ion chamber instruments. When used for gamma radiography, GM meters are typically calibrated for the energy of the gamma radiation being used.

Advantage: It is relatively low cost and rugged. The disadvantages of GM survey meters are the lack of ability to account for different amounts of ionization caused by different energy photons and need to discharge.

T ROD (Fig. 20.11)

It is used to secure the source in its fully shielded position while the cobalt unit is off. In the unlikely event of source drawer system failure, to return the source to its fully shielded position. It has three color

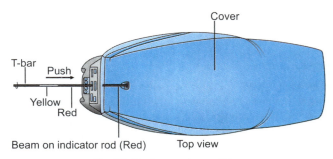

Fig. 20.11 Source drawer T-bar

codes indicative of exact location of source. When the yellow colored portion of the T-bar is entirely inside the head cover, the source is in fully shielded position. If amber-colored portion of the T-bar is visible and the red colored portion is entirely inside the cover, radiation is in the relatively safe level.

Steps to be followed in case of source drawer system failure:

- Open the door and observe the front of the head, if the red tip of the source drawer position indicator rod is visible, high radiation fields will be present in treatment zone and adjoining area.
- Obtain emergency T-bar from its location at console, enter room avoiding exposure in the primary treatment beam.
- Insert the end of the T-bar over the red indicator rod and through the head cover. If the indicator rod is not visible, insert the T-bar through the cover opening until it is felt to engage the indicator rod.
- Apply firm pressure the T-bar and push the source back into fully shielded position. Align the hole in the T-bar with the hole in the cover and insert the locking pin.

Shield

It is a beam modification device. It is used for protection of critical organs, avoiding unnecessary irradiation of surrounding normal tissues and matching adjacent fields.

Properties of ideal shielding material.
- High atomic number
- High density
- Easily available
- Inexpensive.

Ideal shielding material for photons is lead.

Thickness of lead required for shielding in different energies.

Photon energy	Lead thickness
1.25 MV	5 cm
4 MV	6 cm
6 MV	6.5 cm
10 MV	7 cm

Custom Block

It is a beam modification device.

Material used is Lipowitz material, also called Ostalloy Wood's metal.

Composition

- Bismuth   50%
- Lead   26.7%
- Tin   13.3%
- Cadmium   10%

Properties

- Melting point 70 degrees
- Density 9.4 g/cm^3
- Thickness of cerrobend blocks required to produce same attenuation as lead-1.21 times
- Attenuation capability-85% of lead
- Reduces transmission of primary beam to < 3.5%.

Wedge

It is a beam modification device that causes progressive decrease in intensity across beam, resulting in tilting of isodose curves from their normal position.

Properties

Degree of tilt depends on the slope of the wedge filter. Tilt of the isodose curve is toward the thin edge.

It is mounted on the trays at the head of the gantry at a distance of at least 15 cm from skin surface, so as to maintain skin sparing effect.

The material is not of much significance as no hardening is required. Denser material is preferred due to thinner filter size. Commonly used materials are lead, steel tungsten and brass.

The wedges are specified by wedge angle—which is complement of angle through which isodose curve is tilted with respect to the central ray of beam at specified reference depth. Depth is usually taken at 10 cm.

Hinge angle is the angle between the central ray of two intersecting beam.

Bolus

It as a tissue equivalent material placed directly on skin surface to even out irregular contour of patient to present a flat surface on which beam is incident.

Properties

- The electron density, physical density and atomic number should be identical to water, to achieve similar depth dose distribution.
- It should be pliable.
- Specific gravity: 1.02–1.03.

Materials Used

- Slabs of paraffin wax
- Cotton soaked in water
- Mixture D
- Timex rubber
- Lincolnshire bolus-composed of 87% sugar and 13% $MgCO_3$. In form of spheres of ¼ mm diameter contained in linen bags.
- Spier's bolus—composed of 60% rice flour and 40% sodium bicarbonate powder mixture.

Compensator

Beam modifying device that evens out skin surface contour while retaining skin sparing advantage of megavoltage radiation. It allows application of normal depth dose data for irregular surfaces. It provides the required beam attenuation that would otherwise occur in missing tissue when body surface is irregular.

Index

Page numbers followed by *f* refer to figure and *t* refer to table